The Marlowe Diabetes Library

Good control is in your hands.

SINCE 1999, Marlowe & Company has established itself as the nation's leading independent publisher of books on diabetes. Now, the Marlowe Diabetes Library, launched in 2007, comprises an ever-expanding list of books on how to thrive while living with diabetes or prediabetes. Authors include world-renowned authorities on diabetes and the glycemic index, medical doctors and research scientists, certified diabetes educators, registered dietitians and other professional clinicians, as well as individuals living and thriving with prediabetes, type 1 or type 2 diabetes. See page 241 for the complete list of Marlowe Diabetes Library titles.

Gary Scheiner, MS, CDE, is a certified diabetes educator, exercise physiologist, and nutrition consultant who has written dozens of articles and two books on diabetes, fitness, and motivation. He serves on the board of directors of the Diabetes Exercise and Sports Association, and volunteers for the Juvenile Diabetes Research Foundation, American Diabetes Association, and Setebaid Diabetes Camping Services. Drawing upon both his professional skills and personal experience with type 1 diabetes, he teaches the art and science of carbohydrate gram counting and diabetes management to clients throughout the world from his private practice, Integrated Diabetes Services, in Wynnewood, Pennsylvania and through his Web site, www.integrateddiabetes.com.

ALSO BY GARY SCHEINER

*Think Like a Pancreas: A Practical Guide to
Managing Diabetes with Insulin*

THE ULTIMATE

guide to accurate CARB counting

GARY SCHEINER, MS, CDE

Da Capo
LIFE
LONG

A Member of the Perseus Books Group

Designed by Pauline Neuwirth, Neuwirth & Associates, Inc.

Set in 11.5 point Whitman by the Perseus Books Group

Cataloging-in-Publication data for this book is available from the Library of Congress.

ISBN: 978-1-56924-274-2

Published by Da Capo Press

A Member of the Perseus Books Group

www.dacapopress.com

Da Capo Press books are available at special discounts for bulk purchases in the U.S. by corporations, institutions, and other organizations. For more information, please contact the Special Markets Department at the Perseus Books Group, 2300 Chestnut Street, Suite 200, Philadelphia, PA, 19103, or call (800) 810-4145, ext. 5000, or e-mail special.markets@perseusbooks.com.

10 9 8 7

To MJ, Bumblebee, Spiderman and the Princess;
and Debbodil, who makes everything possible.

CONTENTS

WHEN I WAS a kid, my favorite TV character was "the Count" from *Sesame Street*. Sure, his Romanian accent and entourage of bats were pretty neat. But what I really liked was how he made numbers so much fun. Who else could find such joy in counting pumpkins or claps of thunder or whatever else happened to be around? Simply put, the Count made counting cool.

When we become grown-ups, counting is serious business. Why else would we need so many *accountants*? We count how much money we have (or owe), how many miles we get per gallon, how many minutes have passed since the last contraction (as a father of four, I've been there!), how much we weigh, and even the occasional blessing.

There are many counting systems that allow us to monitor and manage our food intake: **Calorie** counting, fat gram counting, point systems, **exchange systems**, and so on. Today, one of the most popular counting system is

carbohydrate gram counting, or **carb counting** for short. And for good reason. Carb counting is important for people with diabetes. It helps those with Type 2 diabetes to control their after-meal blood sugar levels, and it allows those with Type 1 diabetes to match their insulin doses to the amount of carbohydrates consumed. It also has the potential to promote both short-term and long-term weight loss. Many diet plans, including the Atkins, South Beach, and Zone diets, require careful control of carbohydrate intake. Carb counting is important for those who suffer from (reactive) **hypoglycemia** to help minimize the frequency and severity of low-blood-sugar events. Athletes often count carbs to prepare for and excel in competitive events, and managing carb intake has been shown to improve **cholesterol** and **triglyceride** levels.

With so many important uses for carb counting, it seems that everyone should be born with an innate ability to count carbs . . . or at least a guidebook on how to do it right. That's the purpose of this book. It's not to promote any particular approach to managing weight, blood sugars, cholesterol, or energy levels. You and your health-care team are intelligent enough to figure that out. The purpose of this book is to help you to become a more *accurate* and intelligent carb counter. The tools presented in the pages that follow will make carb counting a practical and effective process.

Research presented at the American Diabetes Association annual Scientific Sessions in 2004 showed that even well-managed individuals with type 1 diabetes have difficulty counting carbs accurately, with a tendency to *underestimate* the carbs consumed at breakfast, dinner, and snacks, and *overestimate* the carbs consumed at lunch. A major reason for this is our inability to accurately assess our ever-changing portion sizes. The estimation of complex meals, including restaurant food, is the least precise. Also, meals prepared from scratch using fresh, nonlabeled ingredients can be particularly challenging.

At my own practice, patients who are already experienced carb counters struggle to come up with correct answers to half of the self-test questions scattered throughout this book. With additional training and education, those same patients become proficient at counting carbs accurately.

So let's not waste any more time. Take things at your own pace, enjoy the learning process, and above all, let's make The Count proud!

1

MEET THE CARBS

IT'S TIME FOR some introductions! **Carbohydrates** (or "carbs" for short) are carbon-based molecules that serve as the primary energy source for our body's cells. **Simple sugars, starches,** and **fiber** are all types of carbohydrates, just like cars, buses, and planes are all forms of transportation.

— simple sugars —

Simple sugars are like passenger cars on a highway—they are relatively small, fast-moving, and can be quite stylish (or in this case, tasty!). Most cars on the highway also have only one or two passengers on board. Similarly, simple sugars contain only one or two sugar molecules and are digested easily. Simple sugars include:

- **Glucose** (a building block for starches and other complex carbohydrates), also used in syrups and baking sweeteners. It is present in most fruits.
- **Fructose** (fruit sugar), found in vegetables and fruit, as well as honey and other plant-based sweeteners.
- **Galactose** (combined with glucose to form lactose), rarely found on its own.
- **Dextrose** (also known as corn sugar), used in many cookies, candies, sports drinks, crispy snacks (including dried vegetable chips), and low blood sugar treatments.
- **Lactose** (milk sugar, also found in some plants), present in all cow's milk products and derivatives (milk, butter and most margarines, cheese, condensed and evaporated milk, cream and sour cream, yogurt, ice cream and sherbet, whey) as well as in foods whose ingredients include milk products, such as cream-style soups, most baked goods, and most chocolates. "Lactose-free" soy products are technically dairy lactose free yet may contain the plant form of lactose. Traces of lactose are also found in sourdough breads, soy sauce and miso, green olives, sauerkraut, packaged quick-cook Asian noodles, and salad dressings, as well as some jams and jellies.
- **Sucrose** (derived from cane and/or beets), also known as "table sugar." Aside from being the granulated or cube sugar commonly stirred into beverages, it is used in countless products to add sweetness, color, moisture, and/or tenderness.

- **Maltose** (malt sugar, derived from barley), found in beer, malt whiskey, and other malt beverages, as well as sweetened "natural" foods, malted milk and malted milk–flavored candies, most brands of pretzels, and in the glaze of some Asian dishes.

Sometimes, simple sugars are found in or combined with other substances or flavors, and are listed on ingredient labels as:

- High-fructose corn syrup
- Invert sugar syrup
- Molasses, treacle, and other cane syrup
- Barley malt
- Brown sugar
- Honey
- Maple syrup (also known as pancake or table syrup) and maple sugar
- Sorghum syrup
- Palm sugar
- Agave syrup
- Date sugar
- Brown rice syrup
- Sucanet (as its name suggests, this is largely sucrose)

Even foods you don't think of as being sweet may contain these additives. Some breads contain honey, and most contain some high-fructose corn syrup.

You may have noticed that many "natural," and "sugar-free" products and recipes include these sweeteners. "Natural" though they may be, as compared with highly processed table sugar, *they are still sugar.* Maple syrup, for example, is sucrose, plus a little fructose. Honey may contain nearly two dozen kinds of sugar, with fructose and glucose leading the list. (There are some genuinely sugar-free sweeteners, which I'll get into later. If you can't wait, jump to page 223.)

But we're not done yet—there is also a group of simple sugars called "sugar alcohols," which are simple sugars with a slightly different chemical structure. Some fruits contain trace amounts of sugar alcohol naturally. In most cases, sugar alcohols are synthetic substances produced by food manufacturers to add sweetness to reduced-calorie foods. They do not have the same characteristics as alcoholic beverages, and will not make you drunk! However, they can have a laxative effect, especially when consumed in large quantities. The benefit of sugar alcohols is that they have a sweet taste but digest more slowly and less completely than other simple sugars, providing fewer calories and having less impact upon blood glucose levels than the sugars listed previously. They include:

- ❑ **Sorbitol (**derived from certain fruits; also found in seaweed and algae)
- ❑ **Maltitol** (a modified version of maltose)
- ❑ **Lactitol** (a modified version of lactose)
- ❑ **Mannitol** (derived from algae and fungi such as mushrooms)
- ❑ **Xylitol** (derived from vegetables and fruits)
- ❑ **Erythritol** (derived from fruits)
- ❑ **Isomalt** (a modified version of sucrose)
- ❑ **Hydrogenated starch hydrosylates (HSH)** (converted from starch)

Them's a lot of simple sugars to try to remember! The important thing to keep in mind is this:

> Simple sugars are converted into glucose during the digestive process.

Think of glucose as the gas that drives your car. There are many types of fossil fuel, but we can't take crude oil out of the ground and put it into our cars. It must first be refined and turned into a form that can be accepted and used by an engine. Glucose is the form of energy that is preferred by our body's cells.

Glucose is absorbed into the bloodstream through the walls of the small intestine. Once in the bloodstream, glucose has one of three fates, depending on the body's immediate energy needs: it can (with the assistance of insulin) enter bodily cells to be burned for energy, enter muscle or liver cells for storage (in a dense form called "**glycogen**"), or enter fat cells for conversion to fat (see figure 1).

Simple sugars are only one of the sources of glucose for fueling our body's cells. Let's turn our attention to another important energy source: Starch.

— starch —

Starch is like a bus—it is fairly large and carries many individual passengers that can easily get off when they reach their destinations.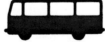
Starches are made up of clusters of glucose molecules,

loosely linked together. Because of the complexity of their structure, they are called **complex carbohydrates**.

Enzymes in the saliva and small intestine break the links holding starches together to produce batches of individual glucose molecules. As was the case with simple sugars, the glucose molecules then absorb through the intestines and circulate in the bloodstream until being taken up by the body's cells.

Some complex carbohydrates/starches are "straight chains" of glucose molecules, like the line of cars that make up a train (see below):

G-G-G-G-G-G-G-G-G-G-G-G-G-G-G

Straight-chain starches are found in many forms of pasta, long-grain rice, and legumes (beans, peas, lentils, peanuts, sprouts, and soy). They break down into glucose slowly because they pack together tightly in bunches.

Others "branch out" at odd angles like the limbs on a tree (see below):

Branched-chain starches are found in most cereals, breads, potatoes, and sticky rice. Because they don't pack together tightly, digestive enzymes have easy access to them. As a result, branched-chain starches convert to individual glucose molecules rather quickly.

Major sources of starches include:

- Wheat
- Rice (all varieties)
- Corn
- Oats
- Rye
- Barley
- Buckwheat
- Millet
- Teff
- Quinoa
- Amaranth
- Triticale
- Kamut
- Spelt
- Sorghum
- Seeds and nuts
- Bananas and plantains
- White potatoes, sweet potatoes, and yams
- Parsnips and carrots
- Carob
- Jerusalem artichoke (also known as sunchoke)
- Cassava (also known as yucca or manioc)
- Jicama (believe it or not, in the bean family)
- Taro (used in Asian/Asian-style cooking and some varieties of Terra snack chips)
- Arrowroot (usually used as a thickener, and in some Asian noodles)

- ❏ Tapioca (dried cassava) and sago (used in desserts and drinks)
- ❏ The following gelling/thickening agents: agar (from seaweed), carrageenan (from algae), kudzu (from a starchy root), guar gum (from the cluster bean), locust bean gum, gum tragacanth (also legume-derived), and xanthan gum (made from corn sugar)
- ❏ Legumes (beans, peas, lentils, soy, peanuts, sprouts)

Be aware that the ever-versatile soy may turn up in foods in the form of tofu, miso, tempeh, soy sauce (which may also contain wheat) and tamari, edamame, soy milk, and other nondairy milklike products such as margarines and cheeses, and soy flours. If you are heavily into natural or Asian foods, you may be consuming way more carbohydrates than you realize!

— simple vs. complex carbs —

How can you tell if a food is rich in simple or complex carbohydrates? Which foods contain both? Be careful when reading only the large print on packaging: some may claim to be "low-sugar" or "low-carb," but such terms may not give you the entire picture. For example, a beer may have a low malt content and yet contain corn or other starchy grains to make up for it.

Again, keep in mind that virtually *every* sugar or starch in a food or beverage will be converted by your body to glucose.

Foods rich in sugar (simple carbohydrates)	Foods rich in starch (complex carbohydrates)
Fruit	Bananas and plantains
Fruit juice, drinks, and punch	Potatoes, sweet potatoes,
Raisins/other dried fruit	and yams
Carrots, beets, and parsnips	Corn
Regular soda	Rice
Cake, pie, pastries, muffins,	Noodles/pasta
and cookies	Cereal
Candy and chocolate	Oats
Milk and milk products	Bread, bagels, and rolls
Ice cream, ices, frozen yogurt,	Soybeans and soy products
and	Crackers
nondairy frozen confections	Crunchy snacks such as
Yogurt	pretzels, chips, and
Beer, malt drinks, and malt	popcorn
whiskey	Pizza
Wine	Tortillas and wraps
Sports drinks	Pancakes and waffles
Granulated, cubed, and pow-	Legumes (peas, beans, and
dered sugar	peanuts)
Brown sugar and molasses	Seeds and nuts
Honey	Beer
Maple and other syrups	Aspics, jelled desserts, and
Jelly, jam, and preserves	puddings
Puddings	

— The "Fate" of Dietary Carbohydrates—

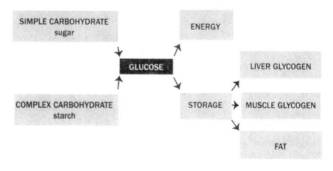

FIGURE 1: Simple and complex carbohydrates are converted into glucose, which is used for energy or stored for future use.

— fiber —

Fiber is a special type of complex carbohydrate. Unlike starches, which break down into simple sugar molecules, the links that hold fiber together are very strong and cannot be broken by the body's digestive enzymes and acids. Think of fiber as a plane: once you get on, you are packed in with lots of other passengers, and you don't get off the plane until you arrive at the final destination. With fiber, that final destination is . . . how shall I put this . . . the toilet. That's right. Fiber passes clear through your digestive system unchanged and is simply pooped away. Its calorie content and contribution to blood sugar levels is insignificant.

Fiber comes in two forms: **soluble fiber**, found in many fruits and vegetables, which dissolves during digestion but remains thick and gummy, and **insoluble fiber**, found in whole grains and legumes, which does not digest at all.

Dietary fiber has a number of important benefits. Because it retains its "bulk" as it moves through the digestive system, it creates a sense of fullness and satiety. This can be very helpful to those who want to control their appetite. In the large intestine, fiber helps make bowel movements softer and bulkier. Fiber tends to absorb toxins that build up in the large intestine, and carries them out of the body. This reduces the risk of several forms of cancer. The same thing happens with cholesterol—fiber prevents the body from absorbing some dietary cholesterol. Fiber also slows the digestive process. This can be helpful in the management of blood glucose levels after meals, since blood sugars rise more slowly when fiber is present.

Unfortunately, the majority of foods in our modern diet have little or no fiber. Processed foods tend to have less fiber than fresh foods. The effect of cooking on the fiber content of foods is unclear; some foods will lose fiber content during the cooking process, whereas others may actually increase. Good fiber sources include:

- Whole-grain cereals
- Whole-grain breads
- Beans and peas
- Oats
- Barley
- Whole, fresh fruit
- Raw vegetables
- Nuts and seeds

Techniques for factoring fiber into carb counts will be discussed in detail in chapter 2. I have also gone to *painstaking* means to include the fiber content along with the carb listings in Tool Kit 4, so make good use of them!

— glycerine —

Glycerine is kind of like a flying saucer. It's there, but not really.

Also known as **glycerin** or **glycerol**, glycerine is derived from triglycerides and is found in some processed diet foods. Although glycerine contains 4 calories per gram, the same as carbohydrates, it does not affect blood sugar levels. However, because glycerine has many of the same chemical properties as carbohydrates, it is included in the total grams of carbohydrates on food labels. If you are counting carbs for weight control, glycerine counts as much as any carbohydrate. But if you are counting carbs purely for blood sugar control, you can take the government's approach to UFOs and act as though glycerine just doesn't exist.

test your carb basics skills

Q: True or False: Sugar alcohols do not raise blood sugar.

A: False—Don't be fooled by misleading product labels. All sugar alcohols raise blood sugar, just not as much as ordinary sugars and more slowly than most other types of carbohydrates.

Q: True or False: Sugar usually has a similar impact on the body as starch.

A: Yes, indeedy. Sugars (simple carbohydrates) and starches (complex carbohydrates) have the same calorie content per gram, raise blood sugars equally per gram, and digest at similarly quick rates.

Q: Carbohydrates include:

   a. Sugars, fats, and starch
   b. Sugar alcohols, starch, and protein
   c. Sugars, fiber, and starch
   d. Sugar, fat, and protein

A: c.—Fat and protein are not carbohydrates. To complete the list, in addition to sugars, fiber, and starch, carbohydrates also include sugar alcohols and glycerine/glycerol.

BASIC CARB-COUNTING TECHNIQUES

I **LOVE THE TV** show *Seinfeld*. In one of my favorite episodes, Jerry Seinfeld is at the airport and goes to pick up a car he reserved at a rental car company. Unfortunately, the company has rented out all of their cars, and Jerry is stuck with nothing to drive. "But I had a reservation," he pleads to the woman at the counter. "I should have a car. That's what reservations are for."

"I know why we have reservations," the woman says.

"I don't think you do," replies Jerry. "If you did, I would have a car. Anyone can *take* reservations. That's easy. What you didn't do is *hold* the reservation, and that's really the most important part of the reservation. *Anyone* can *take* them."

Now, think of Jerry's dilemma in carb-counting terms. Anyone can *count* carbs. (Hey!—there goes one. Here comes another—that makes two!) But not everyone can count carbs *accurately*. And *accuracy* is really the most important part of the carb-counting process. It is what makes your dietary plan **work** for you.

So how do we go from being a carb-counting *guesser* (a reservation "taker") to a carb-counting *expert* (a reservation "holder")? For starters, let's make sure we're all talking the same language. Carbs should be counted in *grams.* Not exchanges or choices. Not ounces or points or drachmas or any other units you might come across. Grams and only grams. Any other method makes carb counting *more* complex and *less* accurate. Grams are the unit of weight used throughout 95 percent of the modern world. Grams are part of the metric system of measurement, which is a much more logical system than the traditional American standards of ounces/pounds, cups/quarts/gallons, inches/feet/yards, and so on. Everything in the metric system is based on the decimal system, which means "ten": units of 10, 100, and 1,000. For example, there are exactly 1,000 micrograms in a gram, and 1,000 grams in a kilogram.

When learning to count carbs, it is best to start simple and become progressively more sophisticated, sort of like learning to add and subtract before diving into algebra. The techniques for counting carbs, ranging from simple to sophisticated, are as follows:

1. Food type (exchange) converting
2. Reading food labels
3. Using nutrient directories
4. Applying food weight/carbohydrate factors
5. Converting portion sizes to carb grams

In this chapter, we'll cover the first three. They are techniques you can master with just a little bit of practice. In the next chapter we'll work on the last two. So let's get started!

— exchange conversion —

One of the most basic methods for counting carbs is a conversion of food categories to grams of carbohydrate. This system is based on the diabetic **exchange system**, whereby foods are grouped according to their typical food content. For example, a slice of bread is equal to a "starch." A piece of fruit is a "fruit."

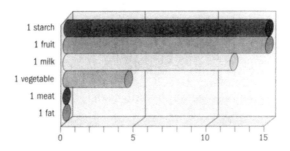

For a complete food category "exchange" list, see Tool Kit 1.

One "Starch" exchange is counted as *15 grams* of carbohydrate. Examples of foods that equal one "Starch" include:

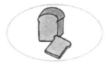

- ❏ 1 slice of bread
- ❏ ½ hamburger bun or English muffin
- ❏ 1 small tortilla or pancake
- ❏ ½ cup of cereal or cooked pasta
- ❏ ⅓ cup of cooked rice or beans

- ❑ ½ cup of peas or white (not sweet) potato
- ❑ ½ medium-size white (not sweet) potato
- ❑ 3 cups popcorn
- ❑ 2 rice cakes
- ❑ 6 saltine crackers
- ❑ 1 small dinner biscuit or regular waffle

One "Fruit" exchange is also counted as *15 grams* of carbohydrate. Examples include:

- ❑ 1 medium-size whole fruit, such as an apple or an orange
- ❑ ½ medium-size banana
- ❑ 1 cup of berries or melon
- ❑ ½ cup of fruit juice

One "Milk" exchange is counted as *12 grams* of carbohydrates. Examples include:

- ❑ 1 cup of milk
- ❑ ⅔ cup of yogurt
- ❑ ⅓ cup of ice cream

One "Vegetable" exchange is counted as *5 grams* of carbohydrate. Examples include:

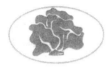

- ❑ ½ cup of cooked, nonstarchy vegetables, such as steamed broccoli, creamed spinach, mashed carrots, or stir-fried zucchini.
- ❑ 1 cup of raw/salad vegetables

All "Meat" (plus cheese and eggs) is counted as *0 grams* of carbohydrate. Examples include:

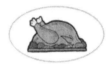

- ❑ beef
- ❑ pork
- ❑ veal
- ❑ lamb
- ❑ poultry
- ❑ fish and shellfish
- ❑ cold cuts
- ❑ cheese
- ❑ eggs

All "Fat" is also counted as *0 grams* of carbohydrates. Examples include:

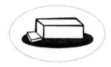

❑ cooking oil
❑ nuts
❑ butter/margarine
❑ sour cream
❑ dressings

To summarize:

> 1 "Starch" = 15 grams carb
>
> 1 "Fruit" = 15 grams carb
>
> 1 "Milk" = 12 grams carb
>
> 1 "Vegetable" = 5 grams carb
>
> 1 "Meat" = 0 grams carb
>
> 1 "Fat" = 0 grams carb

For example, a meal consisting of a sandwich, a small salad with dressing, and a medium-size apple would be counted as follows:

Food Item	Exchange Group/Qty.	Calculation	Carbs for Item
Bread from sandwich	2 starches	2 × 15 g	30 g
Cold cuts	1 meat	1 × 0 g	+ 0 g
Small salad	1 vegetable	1 × 5 g	+ 5 g
Dressing	1 fat	1 × 0 g	+ 0 g
Apple	1 fruit	1 × 15 g	+ 15 g
		Total for meal:	50 g

A meal consisting of a bowl (1 cup) of cereal with ½ cup of milk, 1 cup of orange juice, and 3 strips of bacon would be counted as follows:

Food Item	Exchange Group/Qty.	Calculation	Carbs for Item
Cereal	2 starches	2 × 15 g	30 g
Milk	½ milk	½ × 12 g	+ 6 g
Orange juice	2 fruits	2 × 15 g	+ 30 g
Bacon	3 fats	3 × 0 g	+ 0 g
		Total for meal:	66 g

Using the chart below, try figuring the total carbs for the food items listed. You may refer to Tool Kit 1 in the back of this book for assistance.

Food Item	Exchange Group/Qty.	Calculation	Carbs for Item
Hamburger			
Hamburger bun			
Small (1 cup) fries			
Milk (1 cup)			
1 medium banana			
		Total for meal:	

Using the chart below, try figuring the total carbs for a meal you had earlier today:

Food Item	Exchange Group/Qty.	Calculation	Carbs for Item
		Total for meal:	

The advantage to using the "exchange" system to count carbs is that it is fast and basic. Just about anyone can look at a food item and decide whether it most closely resembles a starch, a fruit, milk, vegetable, meat, or fat, and easily convert those exchanges into a number of grams of carbohydrate. The major problem with this system is that it can be very inaccurate. Portion sizes and food composition can vary considerably, and it is difficult to convert most foods into an exact *number* of exchanges. Even a trained expert would have a hard time figuring out how many starch exchanges are in a bagel just by looking at it. And who really wants to memorize the number of grapes in a fruit exchange?

It also takes considerable guesswork to figure the types and numbers of exchanges in a complex food item such as pizza or soup. Nevertheless, for those who are new to the concept of carb counting, placing foods into their "exchange" category and then converting the exchanges into grams of carb is a natural place to start.

test your exchange system skills

Q: True or False: Most vegetables contain no carbohydrates.

A: False—Just about all vegetables contain *some* carbohydrates. Starchy vegetables (potatoes, corn, peas, etc.) contain 30 to 40 grams of carbohydrate per cup. Non-starchy/salad vegetables (cucumber, tomato, broccoli, spinach, etc.) contain about 5 to 10 grams of carb per cup.

Q: True or False: Half a cup of raisins has more carbohydrate then half a cup of grapes.

A: True—A cup of dried fruit is generally higher in carbohydrates than a cup of fresh fruit because of the fruit's reduced size. There are a lot more raisins than grapes in one cup! Remember: only water is removed during the drying process, not the sugar. In this example, a cup of raisins contains about 100 grams of carb, whereas a cup of grapes has 20 to 25 grams.

Q: True or False: A "starch" exchange has the same amount of carbohydrate as a "fruit" exchange.

A: True—What can I say? The types of carbohydrates vary greatly between these two groups, but in the exchange system each is assumed to contain exactly 15 grams of carbohydrate.

Q: The exchange system is based on the assumption that:

    a. Foods of similar portion size contain similar nutrients.

    b. Foods in one exchange group have similar nutrients as foods in another exchange group.

    c. Foods within a single exchange group have similar calorie content.

    d. Foods within a single exchange group have similar carbohydrate content.

A: d.—Despite its many flaws and weaknesses, one thing about the exchange system that remains somewhat useful is the fact that the items within each category have similar amounts of carbohydrate. The "starch" exchanges have about 15 grams, the milks have about 12 grams, and so on. The tricky part is knowing how *much* of a given item makes up a single exchange!

— label reading —

When it comes to carb counting, labels are like your best friend. They may not always be around but, when they are, they make life a lot more pleasant. Labels are perhaps the most useful and technically accurate sources of information for counting carbs.

The U.S. Food and Drug Administration (FDA) requires all packaged and processed foods to list pertinent nutrient information and ingredients. Exceptions include produce items, which are regulated by the U.S. Department of Agriculture, and alcoholic beverages, which are under the direction of the Bureau of Alcohol, Tobacco and Firearms.

Foods produced in the United States must display a label that lists (among other items) the total carbohydrates, grams of sugar, and dietary fiber in a single serving of the food item, along with the **serving size**. Total carbohydrate is always listed below the "sodium" content. Below the total carbohydrates are listed the dietary fiber and sugar content. Although not required, some food manufacturers will list the amount of soluble and insoluble fiber, along with sugar alcohol and "other" carbohydrates (typically starches) below total carbohydrates.

In Canada, two federal departments—Health Canada and the Canadian Food Inspection Agency (CFIA)—share responsibility for the development and enforcement of food-labeling requirements. The Food and Drugs Act regulates food made, sold, or packaged in Canada. The act specifies the information that the product must have on its label, including a list of ingredients, thirteen specific nutrients (including carbohydrates), and the net quantity of the food product, in both English and French.

In the European Union, nutrition labels are not required unless a "nutrition claim" is made on the package or advertising material. Only nutrition claims that relate to energy value, proteins, carbohydrates, fat, dietary fiber, sodium, vitamins, and minerals are permissible. In many European nations, "serving sizes" have been replaced by standard food weight (such as 100 g) or volume (such as 100 ml), so care must be taken when interpreting nutrient information. For example, a label that lists the carbohydrate content as 20 g (in a 100 g serving) may contain considerably more or less than this amount if the serving size is not exactly 100 grams.

Unfortunately, many popular foods are not labeled. Fresh, nonpackaged, and prepared foods such as fruits, vegetables, baked goods, and restaurant items do not usually come with nutrition labeling. For these types of foods, an alternative carb-counting technique should be used. A nutrient guide (described at the end of this chapter) or a portion estimation technique (described in the next chapter) may be your best option for counting carbs in these types of foods. But first, let's stick with the basics:

However else you obtain your nutritional information, when a label is available, use it! It will contain the most accurate picture of what is contained in the product.

Let's take a look at the pertinent information on a food label:

Super-Hyper Sugar Bits

(Please don't look for this at your local grocery store. I invented this product when I was in seventh grade as part of a package design project in art class.)

Nutrition Facts	
Serving Size ¾ cup (1 oz.)	
Servings per Container 8	
Amount Per Serving	% Daily Value*
Calories 140	
Total Fat 2 g	4%
Saturated Fat 0 g	0%
Trans Fat 0 g	0%
Cholesterol 0 mg	0%
Sodium 120 mg	5%
Total Carbohydrate 30 g	10%
Dietary Fiber 3 g	
Sugars 16 g	
Sugar Alcohol 8 g	
Protein 2 g	
* Percent Daily Values are based on a 2,000 calorie diet.	

1. SERVING SIZE

Serving sizes on food labels are not determined randomly. Experts at the FDA have established more than one hundred food categories and determined specific serving sizes based on "amounts normally consumed." If the portion you eat is smaller or larger than a serving size, you will need to adjust the carbohydrate total accordingly. If a serving size is ½ cup and you have 1 cup, you will need to double the carb amount. If a serving is four squares and you have three, you will have to reduce the carb amount by ¾ (take the carb amount in a single serving and multiply by 0.75).

BE CAREFUL ABOUT SERVING SIZES. The FDA's opinion of what a serving should be may not be what you normally consume. For example, earlier today, I was waiting at the airport for a delayed flight (what else is new?). As the hours passed, I became very hungry and wanted to make sure I had something to eat once I got on the plane. The "king size" Snickers bar I bought seemed like the perfect flight companion! The label indicated that it contained only 21 grams of carbohydrate (including 18 grams of sugar). Not bad! Then I checked the serving size: *one-third of the bar*. One-third? (Not two-fifths or four-sevenths?) I can't imagine anyone taking three separate snacks to finish one candy bar. Or worse, sharing it with two friends! Obviously, the king (in king-size) must have a very small appetite.

2. TOTAL CARBOHYDRATE

Eureka! We've discovered carb-counting gold. In one simple number, the total carbohydrate includes everything in the food item that is carbohydrate—complex carbs (starch and fiber) and simple carbs (sugars and sugar alcohols). Remember to look for the number next to that magic little "g" (grams). The percentage (%) that follows it is the government's estimate of how much of your daily recommended food intake is included in a serving of this food item. *The percentage of daily requirements is irrelevant to the carb-counting process.*

simple carbs (sugars, sugar alcohols)

+ complex carbs (starch/other, fiber)

―――――――――――――――――――――――――

= total carbohydrate

Note: As described in chapter 1, it is not usually necessary to look at simple and complex carbs separately. Sugars and starches both become glucose molecules eventually and have the same caloric content and total impact on blood sugar levels.

So, our initial "label reading" is as follows:

total carbs per serving × number of servings = carb count

Using the label above as an example, if you were to have exactly 1 cup of Super-Hyper Sugar Bits, you would be having: 30 g per serving × 1⅓ serving = 40 g carb.

3. SUGAR

As mentioned previously, sugars are small, simple carbohydrates. Virtually all dietary sugars are converted into glucose for circulation in the bloodstream. Sugars include glucose, fructose, galactose, dextrose, lactose, sucrose, maltose, and sweeteners that contain them: high-fructose corn syrup, maple products, molasses, brown sugar, and honey. As noted earlier, sugar alcohols are also a type of simple sugar (and are included in the "sugar" listing in nutritional information), but their effects are different from those of other sugars. Sugar alcohols will be addressed in more detail later on.

Now, before reading this next sentence, you'll have to forget everything your mother, grandmother, neighbor, and favorite TV talk show host have ever told you. Ready?

> When counting carbs, it is *not* necessary to know
> how much sugar a food item contains.

Okay, now relax. Take a few deep breaths and try not to operate any heavy machinery for the next few minutes. Remember, sugars are just a *type* of carbohydrate, and are included in the total carbohydrate listings on the label. Just as ice, snow, and sleet eventually turn into plain old water, all sugars convert into glucose as do starches and other "complex" carbohydrates. This, by the way, is why those supposedly "sugar-free" products and recipes that are free of granulated "table" sugar or high-fructose corn syrup *in favor of honey, maple, syrup, fructose, or molasses* are not sugar free at all! So, all carbohydrates can be treated the same. Isn't that simple?

4. FIBER

Okay, maybe not quite so simple. Fiber is like one of those "rule breakers" that my kids learn about in spelling class. Yes, fiber is a type of complex carbohydrate. And yes, it is included in the total carbohydrate listing. But don't forget . . . fiber is not digested! It's as if your dog ate your car key. The key isn't gone forever . . . you just have to wait a while for, you know. Fiber makes its way out just like the keys do—a bit dirtier than when they went in, but otherwise unchanged. And if it doesn't get digested, should we count it? Heck no! We should only count the carbs that turn into glucose and enter the bloodstream.

So the bottom line is this: we can *deduct* all of the fiber grams from the total carbohydrates. That leaves us with the carbs that actually digest.

Our new label reading equation looks like this:

> (total carbs per serving – fiber grams) × number of servings = carb count

Going back to our original label:

Nutrition Facts

Serving Size ¾ cup (1 oz.)
Servings per Container 8

Amount per Serving	% Daily Value*
Calories 140	
Total Fat 2 g	4%
Saturated Fat 0 g	0%
Trans Fat 0 g	0%
Cholesterol 0 mg	0%
Sodium 120 mg	5%
Total Carbohydrate 30 g	10%
Dietary Fiber 3 g	
Sugars 16 g	
Sugar Alcohol 8 g	
Protein 2 g	

* Percent Daily Values are based on a 2,000 calorie diet.

Since there are 3 grams of dietary fiber, we can deduct them from the total carbohydrate. 30 minus 3 equal 27 grams of "digestible" carbs per serving. If you were to have 1 cup, you would be having:

$$(30\text{ g} - 3\text{ g fiber}) = 27 \times 1\tfrac{1}{3}\text{ servings} = 36\text{ g carb}$$

Keep in mind that the fiber content of most foods is quite small (if there is any at all). Most fruits and vegetables have just a few grams of fiber per serving, but beans and fiber-enriched cereals may have almost half of their total carbohydrate in the form of fiber.

Product packaging may make claims about the fiber content based on the following:

Claim on Packaging	Requirement (per US FDA)
More/Enriched/Added Fiber	At least 2.5 g fiber per serving
Good Source of Fiber	2.5–4.9 g fiber per serving
High/Excellent Source of Fiber	5 or more grams of fiber per serving

5. SUGAR ALCOHOL

There is one more little adjustment we have to make if we're going to get this right. Back in chapter 1, I briefly discussed a special type of simple carbohydrate called "sugar alcohol." Sugar alcohols are types of simple sugar that don't digest like other sugars. These are not sugars found in alcoholic drinks. They are **artificial sweeteners** found in many common foods, such as gum, mints, yogurt, ice cream, cookies, and candy. They typically go by names ending in "ol," such as sorbitol, maltitol, lactitol, mannitol, xylitol, and erythritol. Hydrogenated starch hydrolysates (HSH) and isomalt are also sugar alcohols, even though they do not have the –ol suffix.

The key thing to know is that sugar alcohols digest much more slowly than other carbohydrates, and they only digest partially (see chart).

Common Sugar Alcohols	Calories per gram (sugar contains 4 cal/g)	Typically found in...
Sorbitol	2.6	Sugar-free candies, chewing gums, frozen desserts, and baked goods
Xylitol	2.4	Chewing gum, gum drops and hard candy, pharmaceuticals and oral health products (throat lozenges, cough syrups, children's chewable multivitamins, toothpaste, and mouthwashes)
Maltitol	2.1	Hard candies, chewing gum, chocolates, baked goods, and ice cream
Isomalt	2.0	Candies, toffee, lollipops, fudge, wafers, cough drops, throat lozenges
Lactitol	2.0	Chocolate, some baked goods (cookies and cakes), hard and soft candy, and frozen dairy desserts
Mannitol	1.6	Dusting powder for chewing gum, ingredient in chocolate-flavored coating agents for ice cream and confections
Erythritol	0.2	Bulk sweetener in low calorie foods
Hydrogenated starch hydro-lysates (HSH)	3	Bulk sweetener in low-calorie foods, provide sweetness, texture, and bulk to a variety of sugarless products

On average, sugar alcohol's calorie content and effect on blood sugar levels is about *half* that of ordinary sugars. For this reason, when counting carbs, it is necessary to deduct half of the sugar alcohols from the total carb content of a food. Our new label-reading formula looks like this:

total carbs per serving

− 100% of fiber per serving

− 50% of sugar alcohols per serving

× number of servings

_____

carb count

Back to our example:

Nutrition Facts

Serving Size ¾ cup (1 oz.)

Servings per Container 8

Amount per Serving	% Daily Value*
Calories 140	
Total Fat 2g	4%
Saturated Fat 0 g	0%
Trans Fat 0 g	0%
Cholesterol 0 mg	0%
Sodium 120 mg	5%
Total Carbohydrate 30 g	10%
Dietary Fiber 3 g	
Sugars 16 g	
Sugar Alcohol 8 g	
Protein 2 g	

* Percent Daily Values are based on a 2,000 calorie diet.

Let's assume once again that you are having 1 cup. Since there are 8 grams of sugar alcohol, we can deduct 4 from the total carb count. And since there are 3 grams of fiber, we can deduct all 3 from the total carb count. Our final carb count is:

$$30 \text{ g}$$
$$- 3 \text{ g fiber}$$
$$- 4 \text{ g sugar alcohol}$$
$$\overline{}$$

23 g carb per serving

23 g carb per serving × 1⅓ servings = 31 g carb

Try these examples:

Benny Bites

Nutrition Facts

Serving Size: 1.5 oz. (1 bag)

Servings per Container 1

Amount per Serving

Calories 100

Total Fat 1 g

    Saturated Fat 0 g

    Trans Fat 0 g

Cholesterol 0 mg

Sodium 150 mg

Total Carbohydrate 20 g

    Dietary Fiber 2 g

    Sugars 1 g

        Sugar Alcohol 0 g

Protein 0 g

What is the accurate carb count, if you eat half of the bag of Benny Bites?

Benny Bites: (20 g total carb − 2 g fiber)

$= 18\text{ g} \times 1/2 \text{ serving} = \textbf{9 g carb}$

Jilly Beans

Nutrition Facts

Serving Size 10 beans

Servings per Container 4

Amount per Serving

Calories 40

Total Fat 0 g

    Saturated Fat 0 g

    Trans Fat 0 g

Cholesterol 0m g

Sodium 120 mg

Total Carbohydrate 16 g

    Dietary Fiber 0 g

    Sugars 16 g

        Sugar Alcohol 12 g

Protein 0 g

What is the accurate carb count if you eat 20 beans?

Jilly Beans: (16 g total carb − 6 g sugar

alcohol) $= 10\text{ g} \times 2 \text{ servings} = \textbf{20 g carb}$

Unfortunately, sugar alcohols are not always listed on the food label. The FDA does not require manufacturers to list the sugar alcohols, and some manufacturers choose not to list them separately from other sugars. Perhaps this is because many people choose to avoid foods that contain sugar alcohols since they can cause diarrhea and intestinal discomfort, especially when consumed in large quantities. By "hiding" the sugar alcohols in the ingredient list (and not listing it under the carbohydrate content), some food manufacturers believe that they can avoid scaring off potential consumers.

If a product lists a sugar alcohol in the ingredients list but does not specify *how much* is in each serving, you can calculate the amount based on the other information contained on the food label. Here is how:

1. Compute how many **calories** in the food come from fats, protein, and ordinary (nonfiber) carbohydrates. Fats have 9 calories per gram, whereas protein and ordinary carbohydrates have 4 calories per gram. Add the calories together.
2. Subtract the total calories listed on the food label from the total calories calculated above (from protein, fat, and nonfiber carbs). The result is the calories from sugar alcohol.
3. Divide the calories from sugar alcohol by 2. The result is the approximate grams of sugar alcohol found in a single serving.

For example:

Apple Jackies

Nutrition Facts
Serving Size ¾ cup
Servings per Container 12
Amount per Serving
Calories 64
Total Fat 4 g
Saturated Fat 0 g
Trans Fat 0 g
Cholesterol 0 mg
Sodium 10 mg
Total Carbohydrate 12 g
Dietary Fiber 2 g
Sugars 10 g
Protein 1 g

To figure the amount of sugar alcohol in a serving of this "low-sugar" cereal substitute:

1. Compute how many calories come from everything *except* sugar alcohol.

multiply fat (4 grams) by 9 calories/gram:	(4g × 9 = 36 calories)
multiply protein (1 gram) by 4 calories/gram:	(1g × 4 = 4 calories)
multiple nonfiber carbohydrates (12 – 2 = 10)	
by 4 calories/gram:	(10 × 4 = 40 calories)
total:	36 + 4 + 40 = 80

2. Subtract the calories per serving (found on the label) from the non-sugar-alcohol calories.

80 calories – 64 calories = 16 calories from sugar alcohol

3. Divide the result by 2 to determine the grams of sugar alcohol in the food.

16 calories ÷ 2 calories per gram = 8 grams

Of the 10 grams of sugar contained in a serving of this item, 8 grams are sugar alcohol.

— artificial sweeteners —

Increasingly, food manufacturers are adding artificial sweeteners to food in an effort to improve their appeal to health-conscious consumers. The exact amount of artificial sweetener contained in the food is not typically given, but the names of the sweeteners are provided in the ingredient listings. In most cases, the exact amount is irrelevant, since their calorie and carbohydrate content is insignificant. Examples include:

- ❏ **Aspartame** (NutraSweet, Equal, NatraTaste, InstaSweet)
- ❏ **Acesulfame-K** (Ace-K, Sweet One, Sweet-N-Safe, Sunette)

- ❏ **Saccharin** (Sweet 'N Low, Sugar Twin, Necta Sweet)
- ❏ **Sucralose** (Splenda)

— what about glycerine? —

Glycerine was introduced briefly at the end of chapter 1. Also known as glycerin or glycerol, glycerine is derived from triglycerides (fats) and is found in some "low-carbohydrate" snacks or meal replacement/energy bars. Glycerine adds moisture and some "sweetness" to foods that might otherwise be lacking in these features.

Although glycerine contains four calories per gram, the same as carbohydrate, it does not affect blood sugar levels. However, because glycerine has many of the same chemical properties as carbohydrates, the Food and Drug Administration (FDA) has ruled that glycerine is a carbohydrate and must be added to the total grams of carbohydrate on the label. If present in a food item, glycerine will be listed in the ingredients section of the food label, but its exact amount is typically not listed under the total carbohydrates.

If you plan to consume a food product that contains glycerine, and your primary purpose of counting carbs is to manage blood sugar levels, the grams of glycerine should be subtracted from the total carbohydrate, much in the same way that fiber is deducted. To obtain the exact amount of glycerine, call the product's manufacturer. However, if weight control/calorie counting is your primary objective, the glycerine content should not be deducted since it contributes as many calories as ordinary carbohydrates.

— about food packaging —

Food labels should not be confused with *claims* made on food packaging. Food packaging can sometimes be misleading, as manufacturers reach for ways to entice you to purchase their products. Several years ago, the U.S. Food and Drug Administration stepped in to try to reduce the misrepresentations. For example:

Claim on Packaging	Requirement (per US FDA)
Reduced Sugar	At least 25% less sugar than a normal version of the same product.
Sugar Free	Less than 0.5 g sugar per reference amount and per serving.
No Sugar Added	No simple sugar or sugar-containing ingredient is added during processing. (Note that this only pertains to *added* ingredients. The original food item could still have sugar in it!)
Not a significant source of sugars	Less than 1 g of sugar per serving.
Low Sugar	This is not defined. There is no basis for content or recommended intake.
Light or Lite	At least 33% fewer calories or 50% less fat than a "nonlight" version of the same product.
Not a significant source of dietary fiber	Less than 1 g of fiber per serving.
Net Carbs, Impact Carbs,	These are non-FDA-endorsed listings that appear on some food labels.

Claim on Packaging	Requirement (per US FDA)
Effective Carbs, Net Atkins Count	Typically, they represent the total carbs minus all of the fiber grams, sugar alcohols, and glycerine. Since sugar alcohols contribute to the caloric and carbohydrate content of foods, and glycerine contributes to the caloric content, these terms can be misleading and should not be used as carb-counting tools.

Occasionally, health organizations may offer "endorsement" or allow the manufacturer to place their logo on product packaging. For example, American Heart Association endorsement means that the product meets criteria for low-cholesterol and low saturated fat. It does not imply anything concerning carbohydrate content. The presence of a logo from the American Diabetes Association or another health-promoting organization usually implies that a portion of the product sales are donated to that organization; it does not imply anything about the product's carbohydrate content or health value.

Q: True or False: "Sugar-free" chocolate often has the same total carbohydrate as regular chocolate.

A: True—Don't be fooled by misleading packaging! The *total* carbohydrates (including sugars and sugar alcohols) are about the same in sugar-free and regular chocolate, as well as sugar-free and regular ice cream. However, don't forget that you can deduct half of the sugar alcohols from the total carb count.

Q: Fiber is a unique type of carbohydrate because it:
   a. Does not raise blood sugar or contribute calories
   b. Raises blood sugar half as much as other carbohydrates
   c. Has half as many calories as other carbohydrates
   d. Blocks the absorption of carbohydrates into the bloodstream

A: a.—Yea, Fiber! Fiber has many wonderful benefits, including giving us a sense of satiety (fullness), reducing serum cholesterol levels and colon cancer risk, as well as helping to stabilize blood glucose levels after meals. Because fiber is resistant to our digestive enzymes, it contributes neither calories nor sugar.

Q: Sugar alcohols:
   a. Raise blood sugar half as much as other sugars
   b. Digest more slowly than other sugars
   c. Both a. and b.
   d. Neither a. nor b.

A: **c.**—Sugar alcohols are used as sugar substitutes in many "diet" and "reduced-calorie" foods because they provide sweetness while contributing only half the calories and blood sugar-raising impact as regular sugar. Their rate of digestion is also much slower than most other simple sugars and complex carbohydrates.

Q: According to the nutritional information below, how much digestible carbohydrate is in a 2-cup portion?

    a. 11 g
    b. 12 g
    c. 22 g
    d. 24 g

Nutrition Facts

Serving Size 1 cup
Servings per Container 8

Calories 116	
Calories from Fat	31%
Total Fat 4 g	
Sodium 15 mg	
Potassium 100 mg	
Total Carb 12 g	
Dietary Fiber 0 g	
Sugar 11 g	
Protein 8 g	

A: **d.**—There is no fiber, so all 12 g carb per serving are digestible. Two cups equals two servings, so 2 × 12 = 24.

Q: According to the nutritional information below, how much digestible carbohydrate is in one bar?

    a. 9 g

    b. 14 g

    c. 19 g

    d. 24 g

Nutrition Facts

Serving Size 1 bar

Servings per Container: 6

Calories 130

Calories from Fat   56%

Total Fat 8g

Sodium 20mg

Potassium 40mg

Total Carbohydrate 19g

    Dietary fiber 0g

    Sugar 12g

        Sugar Alcohol 10g

Protein 1g

A: b.—Did you remember to account for the sugar alcohol? There are 10 g of sugar alcohol per bar, so we can subtract 5 g (10 ÷ 2) from the 19 g of total carb. 19 − 5 = 14.

Q: According to the nutritional information below, how much digestible carbohydrate is in one box?

    a. 24 g

    b. 38 g

    c. 42 g

    d. 52 g

Nutrition Facts

Serving Size 1 box

Servings per Container 1

Calories 90	
Calories from Fat	10%
Total Fat 0 g	
Sodium 30 mg	
Potassium 60 mg	
Total Carbohydrates 38 g	
Dietary Fiber 14 g	
Sugar 4 g	
Protein 2 g	

A: a.—Man, that's a lot of fiber! Since we can subtract all of the fiber grams from the total carbs, we only count this as 38 – 14, or 24 grams of carb.

Q: According to the nutritional information below, how much digestible carbohydrate is in a 1½-cup portion?

    a. 14 g

    b. 16 g

    c. 21 g

    d. 24 g

Nutrition Facts

Serving Size 1 cup

Servings per Container 12

Calories 77	
Calories from Fat	12%
Total Fat 1 g	
Sodium 70 mg	
Potassium 120 mg	
Total Carbohydrates 24 g	
Dietary Fiber 8 g	
Sugar 6 g	
Sugar Alcohol 4 g	
Protein 3 g	

A: c.—Give your brain a chance to rest after figuring out this one. Once we deduct half of the sugar alcohol (2 g) and all of the fiber (8 g) from the total carbs, we come up with 14 grams of digestible carb per serving. Since we're having 1½ servings (a serving is 1 cup), we multiply 14 g by 1.5 to get 21 g.

— a guide to nutrient guides — and other resources

As useful as food labels are, they can only help us count carbs if they are present. Unpackaged foods such as fresh fruits and vegetables, bakery items, restaurant/cafeteria foods, and prepared foods from grocery stores typically do not carry a label. For these types of foods, a **nutrient guide** can be extremely useful. A nutrient guide is a printed or electronic listing of the nutrient contents of many foods. Ideally, a listing should include:

- ❏ A realistic serving size
- ❏ Total carbs per serving
- ❏ Grams of fiber per serving (if any)

The fact is, very few nutrient guides contain all of this information. Most include just a generic serving size and total carbohydrates. For your convenience, the second half of this book features a nutrient guide with all of the above items for many common, ethnic, and prepared foods.

Besides the tool kits in this book, there are many pamphlets, books, Web sites, and other resources that list the carbohydrate content of unlabeled foods. Some cover specific categories such as restaurant food or ethnic food, while others cover a wide range of commonly consumed foods.

USEFUL BOOKS

- ❏ *The Doctor's Pocket Calorie, Fat & Carbohydrate Counter* by Allan Borushek. A compact paperback with comprehensive listings of carb content for common foods, ethnic foods, restaurant foods, and beverages. Indexed for easy searching. Available through Integrated Diabetes Services (877-735-3648, www.integrateddiabetes.com) or Family Health Publications (949-642-8500, www.calorieking.com).

❑ *The Stop & Go Fast Food Nutrition Guide* by **Steven G. Aldana, Ph.D.** A guide to nutrient listings (calories, fat, cholesterol, sodium, and fiber) for foods served at more than sixty-five regional and national fast-food restaurant chains.

❑ *Nutrition in the Fast Lane* by **Franklin Publishing.** A slim brochure containing nutritional content for most menu items from dozens of popular restaurant chains. Call 800-634-1993 to order.

❑ *Bowes and Church's Food Values of Portions Commonly Used* by **J. Pennington.** A large nutrient reference guide for thousands of foods, published by Lippincott. Available at most major bookstores and online retailers.

❑ *The Diabetes Carbohydrate and Fat Gram Guide* by **Lea Ann Holzmeister.** Includes carbohydrates and exchanges for many common foods and restaurant items. Contact the American Diabetes Association, 800-232-6733, or visit http://store.diabetes.org.

❑ *The Complete Book of Food Counts* by **Corinne T. Netzer**. Featuring thousands of listings for generic, brand-name, gourmet, health, and ethnic foods. Available through major bookstores, or through the Random House online catalog at

www.randomhouse.com/catalog (search for
ISBN 9780440241232).

❑ *Guide to Healthy Restaurant Eating* by Hope
Warshaw. In addition to providing nutrition
information (carbs, fat, cholesterol, calories) for
the foods sold at dozens of major chain restaurants, this book teaches strategies for meal planning and healthy restaurant eating. Contact the
American Diabetes Association, 800-232-6733,
or visit http://store.diabetes.org.

❑ *Exchange Lists for Meal Planning*. Booklet produced by the American Diabetes Association and
the American Dietetic Association. To order, call
800-232-6733 or visit http://store.diabetes.org

FREE INTERNET-BASED CARB LISTS

❑ www.nal.usda.gov/fnic/foodcomp/search/ is
your portal to the U.S. federal government's
immense nutrient database. It contains thousands of food items with nutrient content
(including total carbohydrates, fiber, and the
quantity of each type of sugar found in many
food items). Information can be displayed based
on a specific volume or weight for each food
item. The database can be downloaded or
viewed on screen.

❑ For chain (convenience) restaurants, simply type
the name of the restaurant into a search engine.
Most companies have their own Web sites with
nutrient listings for their current menus. Be careful to check the specific serving sizes for the

items you are consuming! Examples include:

- **Arby's:** www.arbys.com/nutrition/
- **Boston Market:** www.bostonmarket.com/restaurant
- **Burger King:** www.bk.com/Food/Nutrition/NutritionWizard/index.aspx
- **Dairy Queen:** www.dairyqueen.com/en/US/Menus+and+Nutrition/Nutrition+Charts/default.htm
- **Denny's:** www.dennys.com/en/cms/Nutrition/Allergens/23.html
- **Dunkin' Donuts:** www.dunkindonuts.com/aboutus/nutrition/
- **KFC:** www.kfc.com/kitchen/nutrition.htm
- **McDonald's:** www.mcdonalds.com/usa/eat/nutrition_info.html
- **Old Country/Hometown Buffet:** www.buffet.com/nutritioncontent.htm
- **Pizza Hut:** www.pizzahut.com/menu/nutritioninfo.asp
- **Starbucks:** www.starbucks.com/retail/nutrition_info.asp
- **Subway:** www.subway.com/applications/NutritionInfo/index.aspx
- **Taco Bell:** www.tacobell.com/
- **Wendy's:** www.wendys.com/food/NutritionLanding.jsp

SOFTWARE FOR PCS AND PDAS

❏ **EzManager Plus** from Animas Corporation includes a database of five thousand foods, and features a dosage calculator and meter downloading option for those who use insulin. Also tracks total carbs and daily activities. Use of the Animas insulin pump is not required. Contact Animas at 877-937-7867 or visit www.animascorp.com.

❏ **DiabetesPilot:** Includes a carb-specific database and summing option for meals. Versions for Windows desktop computers, Palm handhelds, and Pocket PC (Windows Mobile) handhelds are available as shareware from www.diabetespilot.com.

❏ **NutriGenie** is an award-winning nutrition software package featuring a database with over eight thousand items, plus the ability to add the user's own foods. Analysis includes carbs and fiber. Visit http://nutrigenie.biz/index.html.

❏ **Calorie King Diet and Exercise Manager** on CD-ROM includes a thirty-thousand-plus item database, including many ethnic, restaurant, and convenience foods. Available through Integrated Diabetes Services (877-735-3648, www.integrateddiabetes.com) or Family Health Publications (949-642-8500, www.calorieking.com).

TEACHING TOOL FOR CHILDREN

❏ HealthSimple, LLC (formerly Carb Cards LLC) has a series of great items. Visit www.health simpletools.com or call 612-874-6735. They include:

1. FlashCarbs are colorful cards that help adults and children to learn the carb counts of common foods. Fifty cards per deck.

2. FlashCarb Magnets are the same as Flash-Carbs but they adhere to the fridge.

3. Carb Count Stickers can be used for labeling leftovers, bag lunch items or any foods that don't come in a package with nutritional information. Pad of 200 stickers.

ADVANCED CARB-COUNTING
TECHNIQUES

— "1 inch equals 8 grams" —
portion guestimation

A highly practical technique for counting carbs is **portion estimation** (or "guestimation"). This method is particularly useful when having complex meals, dining out, or enjoying foods that vary in size.

Portion guestimation involves using a common object such as your fist, a tennis ball, or a milk carton to determine the approximate volume of a food item, and then converting the volume measurement into a carb count based on the typical carb (per unit volume) for that type of food.

Confused? Don't be. Here's an example that should make this very clear: If you know that one cup of fruit juice contains about 30 grams of carbohydrate, and you are having a portion of juice equal to 1½ cups, you are having 30 × 1½, or 45 grams of carbohydrate.

The key to making this method work is to obtain a fairly accurate size estimate for your food portions. Below are some common "measuring devices" that can be used for physically "seeing" or mentally "visualizing" portion volumes:

❏ 12-ounce soda can = 1½ cups

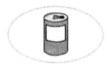

❏ Average adult's fist = approximately 1 cup

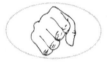

❏ Child's fist = approximately ½ cup
❏ Cupped hand = approximately ½ cup
❏ Large handful = approximately 1 cup

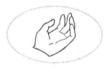

❏ Tennis ball = approximately ¾ cup

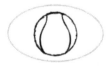

- ½ pint milk = 1 cup
- Deck of cards = approximately ⅓ cup

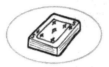

- Adult's spread hand = approximately 8" diameter

- Adult's palm = approximately 4" diameter

When estimating portion volume, it is helpful to have the measuring device right next to the food item. For instance, placing your fist next to a salad will allow you to estimate the number of "cups" of salad. Having a half-pint container of milk or a can of soda next to a plate of spaghetti will allow you to do the same. Keep in mind that *volume* consists of three dimensions: length, width, and *height*. The thickness/tallness of the food item should be taken into account when estimating the volume. Also, be sure to count only the portion that you are actually going to eat. The rind or peel on fruit, for example, should not be counted; nor should potato skins or bread crusts if you don't plan to eat them.

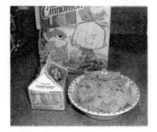

In the picture to the left, it would be difficult to estimate the amount of cereal in the bowl simply by looking at it from the top. Comparing the cereal (which is "topped off" in the bowl) to the ½ pint (1 cup) container of milk, we can tell that there is about 1½ cups of cereal.

In the picture to the right, seeing the apple right next to the can of soda gives us a good view of its actual volume. Given that it is half of the 1½-cup can's size, we can accurately determine that the apple measures about ¾ cup.

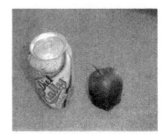

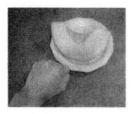

In the picture to the left, we can visualize that the *volume* of the cantaloupe (height included) is slightly more than an adult's fist, or about 1¼ cups.

The best way to fine-tune your portion estimation skills is through practice—practice, practice, and more practice. Estimate the volume of a food item (using your fist or another item of known volume for comparison), and then either look up the exact volume on the food's label or place it in a measuring cup. Doing this repeatedly will train your eye and your mind to estimate portions accurately.

Great. Now you can figure out exactly how many quarter cups there are in a serving of your Aunt Patty's famous potato salad. Where do we go from here?

Easy! Now we turn it into grams of carb!

Below are approximate carb counts for standard portion sizes of many common foods:

Food Type	Specific Items	Approximate Carb Content in 1 Cup (prepared)
Potato	Baked, mashed, scalloped French fries	40 g
Pasta	Spaghetti, linguine, macaroni, ziti, lasagne	40 g
Rice	Instant rice, fried rice	50 g
"Sticky" rice	Steamed/pressure-cooked rice, Asian restaurant rice	75 g
Nonstarchy vegetables (raw)	Mixed salad vegetables, tomato, pepper, carrot, spinach, broccoli, cauliflower	5 g
Nonstarchy vegetables (cooked)	Steamed, stir-fried, boiled, creamed, mashed vegetables such as those listed above	10 g
Corn and peas	Most types/brands	30 g
Beans	Kidney beans, lima beans, butter beans, chickpeas	40 g
Soft breads	Dinner rolls, kaiser rolls, sandwich rolls, buns	25 g
Dense breads	Bagels, soft pretzels	50 g
Fruit (summer)	Berries, melons, peaches, tropical fruit	20 g
Fruit (winter)	Pears, bananas, apples, oranges	25 g
Pastries	Cake, muffin, pie, Danish	50 g

Food Type	Specific Items	Approximate Carb Content in 1 Cup (prepared)
Pretzels and crackers	Packaged pretzels, snack crackers	25 g
Chips	Potato chips, tortilla chips, cheese puffs, pork rinds	15 g
Popcorn	Air popped, microwaved, packaged	5 g
Ice Cream	Ice cream custard, ice milk, frozen yogurt	35 g
Dry cereal	Corn flakes, wheat flakes, crisp rice, Cheerios	25 g
Milk	Regular, skim, 2%	12 g
Juice	Orange, apple, grape	30 g
Sauce	Tomato-based sauces	20 g
Soft drinks	Reg. soda, lemonade, punch	30 g
Sports drinks	Gatorade, Powerade	15 g

grams of carb per cup × number of cups = carb count

Using this approach with a portion of pasta equal to two "fists," there would be 40 g/cup × 2 cups, or 80 grams of carb. Three large handfuls of chips would have 15 g/cup × 3 cups, or 45 g carb.

Returning to the pictures shown on page 58, the 1½-cup portion of cereal flakes equals 25 g per cup × 1½ cups, or about 37 g carbohydrate. (the 1-cup milk serving would be 12 g)

The ¾-cup apple would be 25 g per cup × ¾ cups, or about 19 g carb.

The 1¼-cup piece of cantaloupe has 20 per cup × 1¼ cups, or 25 g carb.

There are a number of other "tricks" for estimating food portions that involve length and surface area rather than volume measurements. For example:

Long sandwiches (sub, hoagie, hero, grinder)	8 g per inch
Sushi (roll or cone)	7 g per piece
Pizza	30 g per adult hand-size piece (fingers together)
Pancakes	20 g per adult hand-size pancake (fingers spread)
Cookies	20 g per adult-size palm
Tortillas	15 g per adult-size hand (fingers spread)
Breaded meats/vegetables/ cheeses	4 g for small piece (thumb-size nugget) 10 g for large piece (palm-size patty)
Syrup	15 g/tablespoon

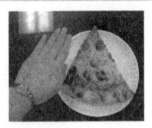

For example, a 6"-long hoagie (can't help it . . . I live in Philadelphia) sandwich contains approximately 8 g/inch × 6 inches, or 48 grams of carb. A slice of pizza a bit larger than an adult's hand (see above) would have approximately 1⅓ × 30, or 40 grams of carbohydrate. Of course, if we were counting for one of my kids, it would be closer to 30 g, since none of them eats the crust. (They usually just toss their crusts onto my plate like throwing bones to a dog. . . . Okay by me—the crust is my favorite part!)

test your guesstimation skills

Q: True or False: A cup of carrots has as many carbohydrates as a cup of potatoes.

A: False—What's the deal, Doc? Carrots have really gotten a bad rap lately! Although higher in sugar content than some vegetables (like lettuce and celery), carrots are still significantly lower in carbs than starchy vegetables like potatoes, peas, and corn.

Q: True or False: A cup of rice usually has more carbohydrates than a cup of pasta.

A: True—There is about 50 grams of carb in a cup of instant rice, and 30–40 grams in a cup of pasta. Rice prepared at most Asian restaurants is even higher—as much as 75 g carb per cup, because the starch that the rice sheds as it cooks is not rinsed off.

Q: Approximately how many grams of carbohydrate are in this portion of salmon with pasta?

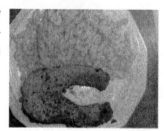

   a. 20
   b. 40
   c. 60
   d. 80

A: c.—Plain pasta contains about 40 grams of carbohydrate per cup. Remember, as a rule of thumb, an average-size adult's fist measures about 1 cup. There is roughly 1½ fist-size portions of pasta on the plate, for a total of 60 grams. The salmon's carbohydrate content is negligible.

Q: Approximately how many grams of carbohydrate are in this soft pretzel?

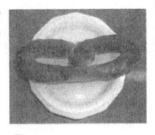

    a. 30

    b. 45

    c. 60

    d. 90

A: c.—Surprising, eh? The average soft pretzel has a little more than a cup of "heavy bread" (at 50 g/cup), so we'll call it about 60. Most bagel-store and bakery bagels have a similar size/quantity of carbohydrate as the pretzel shown in the picture.

Q: Approximately how many grams of carbohydrate are in this tossed salad and diet soda?

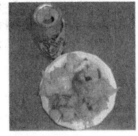

    a. 0

    b. 5

    c. 10

    d. 15

A: b.—Yes, even salad has some carbohydrate. Each cup of mixed raw veggies contains about 5 grams of carbohydrate. Given that this small "side" salad is approximately 1 cup, we're looking at 5 grams of carbohydrate.

Q: Approximately how many grams of carbohydrate are in this portion of cooked mixed vegetables and diet soda?

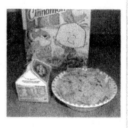

a. 0
b. 5
c. 10
d. 20

A: c.—Once again, there is about a cup of cooked non-starchy vegetable on the plate; each cup contains about 10 grams of carbohydrate.

Q: Approximately how many grams of carbohydrate are in this portion of Life cereal and whole milk?

a. 20
b. 30
c. 40
d. 50

A: d.—8 ounces (1 cup) of milk contains 12 grams of carbohydrate regardless of the fat content (ie., 1%, 2%, skim, or whole). Most cereals provide about 25 grams of carbohydrate per cup. The bowl of cereal is about 1½ times the size of the cup of milk, for 35–40 grams of carb. In this instance, milk + cereal = 50 grams of carbohydrate.

Q: Approximately how many grams of carbohydrate are in these waffles and real maple syrup?

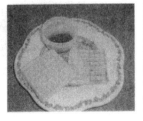

    a. 25

    b. 45

    c. 60

    d. 75

A: b.—Your average garden-variety frozen waffle contains about 15 grams of carb. Real maple syrup contains about 15 grams per tablespoon. The small syrup portion shown here represents about a tablespoon. 15 g + 15 g + 15 g = 45 g.

Q: Approximately how many grams of carbohydrate are in this peach and diet soda?

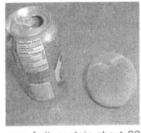

    a. 5

    b. 10

    c. 25

    d. 30

A: b.—Peaches, being a summer fruit, contain about 20 grams of carb per cup. This ½-cup-size peach contains about 10 grams of carb.

Q: Approximately how many grams of carbohydrate are in this portion of chicken breast, cooked carrots, and mashed potatoes?

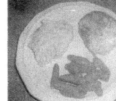

a. 15

b. 20

c. 35

d. 40

A: c.—Baked chicken has no carbs (unlike breaded/fried chicken, which contains 5–15 grams of carb per piece depending on the size). A cup of cooked veggies has about 10 grams, and 1 cup of potato (any form) contains about 40 grams of carbohydrate. Given that this looks like about ¾ of a cup of each, we have 30 grams of potato carb and 5–8 grams of carrot carb for a total of about 35 grams.

Q: Approximately how many grams of carbohydrate are in this portion of popcorn and diet soda?

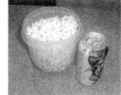

a. 5

b. 20

c. 40

d. 60

A: b.—It looks higher than it actually is! Each cup (or large handful) of popcorn contains only about 5 grams of carb. There are approximately 4 cups of popcorn in the bowl, for a total of 20 grams.

Q: Approximately how many grams of carbohydrate are in this slice of sausage pizza?

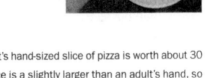

  a. 20

  b. 40

  c. 60

  d. 70

A: b.—An adult's hand-sized slice of pizza is worth about 30 g carb. This slice is a slightly larger than an adult's hand, so go with 40 grams.

— using carb factors —

You might remember *The Odd Couple*, a movie and then a situation comedy about a sloppy, rough-around-the-edges character (Oscar) sharing an apartment with a meticulous, compulsively neat friend (Felix). If the "portion guestimation" technique of carb counting represents the Oscar approach, then the "carb factors" method certainly represents the Felix approach.

Using **carb factors** involves weighing a portion of food on a scale* and then multiplying the weight of the food (in grams) by its carb factor (which represents the *percentage* of the food's weight that is carbohydrate). Doing so will produce a fairly precise carb count for that portion of food.

Food Weight (in grams) × Carb Factor = Carb Count

---

* Food scales can be found at most discount department stores and houseware/kitchenware stores. Be certain to obtain a scale that weighs in grams, and not just ounces. Prices can vary considerably; mechanical "spring" type scales may only cost a few dollars, but they tend to be imprecise (measurement to the nearest 10 or 20 grams), and it can be awkward to fit some foods onto their tray or top. Digital/battery-operated scales vary in price from twenty or thirty dollars (for basic models) to hundreds of dollars (for models that can calculate specific food nutrients based on the food's weight). Digital scales offer the advantages of being very accurate and having a "tare" function (which allows you to factor out the weight of the bowl or plate that the food is on). Personally, I am not a big fan of the expensive "programmable" scales, because they require the user to enter a special code number for each food type before nutrient information can be displayed. In terms of carb counting, if you have to look up a code number, you'd might as well just look up the carb factor and do the math on a calculator! If you are interested in ordering a mechanical or digital scale by mail, feel free to visit my Web site (www.integrateddiabetes.com), or call toll-free, 877-735-3648.

For example, apples have a carb factor of 0.13, which means that 13 percent of an average apple's weight is carbohydrate. If an apple weighs 120 grams, the carb content is 120 × 0.13, or 15.6 grams.

As was the case with portion guestimation, carb factors should only take into account the food that will actually be eaten. Foods should be weighed *without* the peel, rind, skin, seeds, packaging, crust, or any other part that will not actually be consumed. The apple measurement may slightly overestimate the carb count since the core is not usually eaten.

Carb factors are most helpful with foods eaten at home (nobody expects you to carry a scale everywhere you go), where the food may be an odd shape, the density of the food can vary considerably, or the food item is actually a mixture of several foods. Examples include beef stew, homemade breads/pastries and baked potatoes.

A list of carb factors for many common foods is listed in Tool Kit 2, pages 101–107.

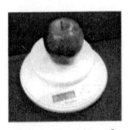 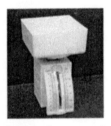

For an alphabetized list of carb factors for more than six thousand foods (in Excel spreadsheet format), go to www.friendswithdiabetes.org/files/Carb factor.xls.

If you tend to take foods out of their packages for storage and won't have a label handy when you consume the food, you should calculate the food's carb factor before the package is discarded. Simply divide the total carbohydrate for a single serving (in grams) by the weight of a single serving (in grams) to derive the carb factor. You can then use the carb factor to calculate the carb content of any size portion when you actually consume it. For example, many people prefer to store noodles in an airtight package rather than in the original bag or box. If the label on the original box indicates the following:

Serving size = 150 g (prepared)

Carb per serving (total carb less 100%

of fiber and 50% of sugar alcohol) = 42 g

The carb factor is 42/150, or 0.28.

If you cook up some noodles and your portion happens to weigh 200 g, you are having 200 × 0.28, or 56 grams of carb.

test your carb factor skills

Q: To calculate grams of carbohydrate based on weight, you would:

   a. Multiply the food's weight (in grams) by its glycemic index
   b. Multiply a food's weight (in grams) by its carbohydrate factor
   c. Multiply a food's weight (in ounces) by its glycemic index
   d. Multiply a food's weight (in grams) by its exchange value

A: b—Carbohydrate factors represent the percentage of a food's weight that is carbohydrate. To get the *grams* of carbohydrate, you must start with the *grams* of food weight, and multiple by its carb factor (found in Tool Kit 2).

Q: How many grams of carbohydrate are in a slice of pumpkin pie weighing exactly 200 grams?

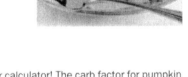

   a. 33 g
   b. 48 g
   c. 62 g
   d. 79 g

A: b.— Get out your calculator! The carb factor for pumpkin pie is .24. Multiply .24 by the weight (200 g), and we get 48 grams of carbohydrate.

Q: How many grams of carbohydrate are in a baked potato weighing exactly 295 grams?

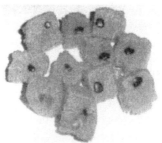

    a. 35 g

    b. 45 g

    c. 65 g

    d. 85 g

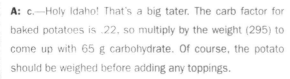

A: c.—Holy Idaho! That's a big tater. The carb factor for baked potatoes is .22, so multiply by the weight (295) to come up with 65 g carbohydrate. Of course, the potato should be weighed before adding any toppings.

Q: How many grams of carbohydrate are in watermelon cubes weighing exactly 300 grams?

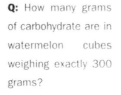

    a. 18 g

    b. 24 g

    c. 30 g

    d. 36 g

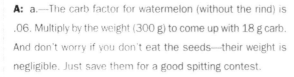

A: a.—The carb factor for watermelon (without the rind) is .06. Multiply by the weight (300 g) to come up with 18 g carb. And don't worry if you don't eat the seeds—their weight is negligible. Just save them for a good spitting contest.

— summary of carb-counting techniques —

	Pros	Cons	Best Used For
Food Group/ Exchange Conversion	❏ Simple ❏ Requires little memorization ❏ Based on common sense	❏ Can be very inaccurate ❏ Is difficult to fit many foods into specific categories	❏ Basic foods only ❏ Beginners
Food Labels	❏ Precise ❏ Easy to interpret	❏ Not all foods are labeled ❏ Foreign labels more difficult to interpret ❏ You must pay careful attention to serving sizes	❏ Packaged foods of any kind
Reference Guides	❏ Simple to use ❏ Easy to find the information you want ❏ Good source of info for complex foods	❏ Listings may not match your food exactly ❏ You need to carry guides with you	❏ Restaurant/ take-out foods ❏ Ethnic foods
Portion Guesstimation	❏ Practical ❏ Convenient ❏ Can apply to virtually any food	❏ Not as precise as labels/ guides ❏ Requires knowledge of carb amount per unit volume ❏ Takes practice to master	❏ Nonpackaged foods ❏ Restaurant/ take-out foods
Carb Factors	❏ Very precise	❏ Requires use of a scale ❏ Need list of carb factors to interpret	❏ Irregular/ mixed/ complex/odd-shaped foods ❏ Foods consumed at home

4

MENU MISCELLANY

YOU COULD HIRE a team of physicists, armed with million-dollar subatomic scales, headed by the head of the dietary department of NASA, and still not get the right carb count for a piece of holiday fruitcake. Sometimes, we just have to learn from our mistakes and do a better job the next time.

Meatballs have always given me personal grief. I love the taste, but the carb counts are not so easy. Some places use a sauce with lots of sugar, some with less. Some places use more bread crumbs than others. Some are denser than others. It's taken some trial and error (and some note-taking) to figure out which places make the lower-carb meatballs, and which places' meatballs could nourish a small city.

In particular, I've found counting the carbs in restaurant food to be particularly challenging. It never hurts to ask the manager if they have a brochure with listings for their menu items. You would be surprised! Most chain restaurants (both sit-down and fast-food) have nutrient listings for at least some of their more popular dishes. Some even post this information at a Web site or in printed form in their lobby or seating areas.

The nutrition guide in this book, as well as many listed earlier in the reference section, can be a tremendous help when eating out. Even if your specific restaurant is not in one of these guides, you can probably find something similar at a restaurant that is in the listings.

Complex recipes can be another source of frustration for carb counters. One way around this is to get a complete list of the ingredients, add up the carbs for everything used in the recipe, and divide by the number of servings. For example, consider the following recipes, taken from the original American Diabetes Association Holiday Cookbook, circa 1986:

— african vegetarian stew —

(serves 8)

INGREDIENTS:

1 whole parsnip

1 large onion

2 sweet potatoes

2 zucchini

1 (16-ounce) can tomatoes

1 (15-ounce can) garbanzo beans

½ cup couscous

¼ cup raisins

1 teaspoon ground coriander

½ teaspoon ground turmeric

½ teaspoon ground cinnamon

½ teaspoon ground ginger

¼ teaspoon ground cumin

3 cups water

To a carb-counting novice, trying to estimate the carbs in African Vegetarian Stew sounds like a daunting task, but it really isn't that difficult. Most of the carbs will be in the potatoes, beans, and couscous, some in the raisins and vegetables, and virtually none in the spices:

2 sweet potatoes (approximately 1 cup each)	80 g
1 (15-ounce can) garbanzo beans (2 cups)	80 g
½ cup uncooked couscous	70 g
1 parsnip	30 g
1 large onion	20 g
2 zucchini	20 g
1 (16-ounce can) tomatoes (2 cups)	30 g
¼ cup raisins	30 g
1 teaspoon ground coriander	0
½ teaspoon ground turmeric	0
½ teaspoon ground cinnamon	0
½ teaspoon ground ginger	0
½ teaspoon ground cumin	0
3 cups water	0

The total is approximately 360 g carb. Since there are 8 servings, each serving would contain about 45 g carb ($360 \div 8 = 45$). If you divide the stew into 10 servings, there would be 36 g carb per serving.

Let's try the same approach with a complex salad dish:

— wild rice waldorf salad —

(serves 4)

INGREDIENTS:

1 cup cooked wild rice

1 apple

1 cup seedless grapes

1 cup celery

2 tablespoons mayonnaise

1 tablespoon plain yogurt

2 tablespoons peanuts

Where would most of the carbs be found in this salad? Definitely in the rice. The fruit would contribute some carbs as well, and the remaining ingredients would contribute very little carbohydrate.

1 cup cooked wild rice	35 g
1 medium apple	20 g
1 cup grapes	25 g
1 cup celery	6 g
2 tablespoons mayonnaise	1 g
1 tablespoon plain yogurt	1 g
2 tablespoons peanuts	4 g

The grand total for the recipe is 92 grams of carb. Divided into 4 portions, that comes to 23 g carb per serving.

Now, how about a nice-a-bowl-a-soupa?

— low-calorie minestrone —

(serves 12)

INGREDIENTS:

8 cups chicken broth

1½ cups chopped celery

1 cup chopped onion

1 zucchini, sliced

2 (16-ounce) cans tomatoes

2 cups finely chopped cabbage

¼ cup chopped fresh parsley leaves

1 garlic clove, minced

1 bay leaf

1 teaspoon dried thyme

½ teaspoon salt

½ teaspoon ground black pepper

Although there are no carb-dense ingredients, there are many items that each contribute small amounts of carbohydrate, with the tomatoes taking the lead:

4 cups tomatoes	40 g (taken from label)
1½ cups celery	9 g
1 cup onion	14 g
1 zucchini	10 g
2 cups cabbage	4 g
8 cups chicken broth	8 g (taken from label)
Misc. other spices	Negligible

The grand total for the recipe is 85 grams of carb. Divided into 12 portions, that comes to about 7 g carb per serving.

No section on menu planning is complete without a tasty dessert. Many people tell me that the word "fruitcake" comes to mind when they meet me, so let's examine one carefully:

— fruitcake —

(serves 15)

INGREDIENTS:

½ cup snipped dried figs

½ cup chopped dates

½ cup chopped prunes

1 cup crushed pineapple

1 cup raisins

2 cups chopped apple

½ cup chopped walnuts

½ cup orange juice

2 cups whole wheat flour

½ cup wheat germ

1 tablespoon baking powder

1 teaspoon ground cinnamon

½ teaspoon ground nutmeg

2 eggs

It appears that most of the carbs are going to come from the fruits (fresh, dried, and juiced) as well as the flour.

½ cup figs	34 g
½ cup dates	57 g
½ cup prunes	28 g
1 cup pineapple	20 g
1 cup raisins	100 g

2 cups apple	50 g
½ cup orange juice	15 g
2 cups whole wheat flour	82 g (112 g minus 30 g fiber)
½ cup wheat germ	18 g (24 g minus 6 g fiber)
1 teaspoon cinnamon	2 g
½ cup walnuts	8 g
1 tablespoon baking powder	1 g
½ teaspoon nutmeg	0 g
2 eggs	0 g

The grand total for the recipe is 415 g, give or take a dried fig. Divided by 15 servings, that comes to 28 g per serving.

test your menu skills

Q: Which meal contains the *greatest* amount of carbohydrates?

    a. 1 cup of sweetened vanilla yogurt and ½ cup of granola

    b. 1 cup frosted flakes and 1 cup whole milk

    c. 1 English muffin with 2 tablespoons peanut butter and 2 teaspoons jelly

    d. 1 cup plain cooked oatmeal with 2 teaspoons butter and 2 teaspoons sugar

A: a.—Sweetened yogurt (yogurt with added sugar and fruit on) contains about 30–40 g/cup. *Believe it or not*, most brands of granola contain about 20 g per ¼ cup. The granola therefore contributes another 40 grams for a grand total of 70–80 g of carbohydrate. Options b., c., and d. each have about 40 grams of carbohydrate.

Q: Which meal contains the *least* amount of carbohydrates?

    a. 1½ cups of brown rice, 12 shrimp, 1 cup of steamed broccoli, and 2 fortune cookies

    b. 10-inch submarine sandwich, and 1 small bag of chips

    c. 1½ cups of pasta with butter, 1 chicken breast, 2 Oreo cookies

    d. 1 cup of potato, ½ cup of peas, 1 dinner roll, a 5 ounce steak, and 1 cup of ice cream

A: c.—This meal totals about 75 grams of carb (60 for the pasta, 0 for the chicken, and 15 for the cookies). Every cup of rice (brown or white) contains about 50 grams carb, a cup of cooked vegetables contains 10, and the cookies are about 10 each, so a. contains about 120 grams of carb. Every inch of submarine sandwich–type bread contains 8 grams of carb, so b. would total about 95 grams (including the chips). Choice d. would have about 105 grams of total carbs: 40 for a cup of potato, 15 for the peas, 15 for an average dinner roll, 0 for the steak, and 35 grams for a typical cup of ice cream.

— enter the 4th dimension —
the glycemic index

Now that you have achieved the rank of Carb Counting Master, it's time for a revelation: Not all carbs are created equal. Another factor that you may want to consider when counting carbs is the influence of the **glycemic index**.

The glycemic index (GI) refers to the rapidity with which carbohydrates convert into blood glucose. While virtually all carbohydrates (except for fiber, glycerine, and a portion of sugar alcohols) convert into blood glucose eventually, some forms convert much faster than others. Pure glucose is given a GI score of 100; everything else is compared to the digestion/absorption rate of glucose. A glycemic index list for many common foods is provided in Tool Kit 3.

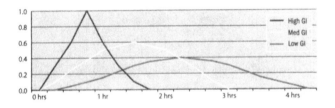

Rates of Carbohydrate Digestion, Relative to the Glycemic Index

Foods with a high GI (greater than 70) tend to digest and convert the fastest, with a significant blood glucose "peak" occurring in 30 to 45 minutes. Examples include bread, potatoes, cereal, and rice. Foods with a moderate GI (approximately 40–70) digest a bit slower, resulting in a less pronounced blood glucose peak approximately one to one and a half hours after eating. Examples include ice cream, orange juice, cake, and carrots. Foods with a low GI (below 40) tend to make a slow, gradual appearance in the blood-stream. Their blood glucose "peak" is usually quite modest, and may take several hours to appear.

High, Moderate, and Low GI Values	
High GI	70 or higher
Moderate GI	41–69
Low GI	0– 40

Fastest	Glucose
	Dextrose
	Starch (branded-chain)
	Sucrose/Corn Syrup
	Fructose
	Starch (straight-chain)
	Lactose
Slowest	Sugar Alcohols

Most starchy foods have a relatively high GI; they digest easily and convert into blood glucose quickly. Exceptions include "straight-chain" starches (see chapter 1) such as those found in pasta and legumes. Because these starches pack together very tightly, digestive enzymes take a while to break them apart—thus causing the slow rate of diges-tion. Foods that have glucose or dextrose in them tend to have a high GI. Fructose (fruit sugar) and lactose (milk sugar) are slower to convert into blood glucose. Table sugar (sucrose) has a moderate GI because it contains a combination of glucose (which is fast) and fructose (which is slow). Foods that contain fiber or large amounts of fat tend to have lower GIs than foods that do not.

Glycemic Index Facts

❏ High-fiber converts slower than low-fiber

❏ High-fat converts slower than low-fat

❏ Solids convert slower than liquids

❏ Cold foods convert slower than hot foods

Why is this important? Because the *effect* of dietary carbohydrates is what really matters. The slower a carbohydrate digests, the less immediate and dramatic its impact will be. Low GI foods tend to make blood sugars easier to control. They enhance satiety and help to curb appetite. They help to lower triglyceride levels and prevent (reactive) hypoglycemia. And they serve as excellent fuel sources in preparation for endurance exercises.

test your glycemic index skills

Q: You can use the glycemic index to help . . .

    a. Figure out the total carbohydrate content of foods

    b. Increase metabolism

    c. Compare the nutritional value of foods within similar categories

    d. Determine the satiety effect of different foods

A: **d.**—The glycemic index describes the speed by which carbohydrate-containing foods convert to glucose in the body. Low glycemic-index foods tend to produce less of a blood sugar "spike" after eating, and a greater sense of satiety (fullness).

Q: Which food should produce the slowest rise in blood glucose?

    a. Pretzels

    b. Corn flakes

    c. Ice cream

    d. Rice cake

A: **c.**—Foods that contain fat and milk sugar (lactose), such as ice cream, tend to convert to glucose slowly. This makes them lower on the glycemic index as compared with grain-based foods, such as cereal and snack foods.

Q: Which food should produce the fastest rise in blood glucose?

   a. Orange juice

   b. Regular soda

   c. Saltine crackers

   d. Chocolate

A: c. Crackers are a high glycemic-index food made of "branched-chain" starches that break down into glucose molecules very quickly. Regular soda, which contains sucrose or high-fructose corn syrup, would also raise blood sugar quickly, but not as fast as the crackers. Orange juice, with fructose as its primary form of carbohydrate, has a lower GI value than crackers and soda, and chocolate (with its high fat content) is slowest of the lot.

tool kits

tool kit 1

AS I **DESCRIBED** in chapter 2, exchange lists are an easy way to categorize foods according to their general nutrient content. For carb-counting purposes, items within an exchange list contain approximately the same amount of carbohydrate.

— starch exchanges —
(approximately 15 g carb per serving)

Cereal/Grains/Pasta

Bran cereals, concentrated	⅓ cup
Bran cereals, flaked (All-Bran Bran Buds, All-Bran)	½ cup
Bulgur, cooked	½ cup
Cooked cereals	½ cup
Cornmeal, dry	1½ teaspoons
Grape-Nuts	3 tablespoons
Grits, cooked	½ cup
Pasta, cooked	½ cup

Rice (white or brown), cooked	½ cup
Shredded wheat	½ cup
Unsweetened cereals	¾ cup
Wheat germ	1 tablespoon

Beans/Peas/Lentils

Lentils, cooked	⅓ cup
Baked beans	¼ cup
Beans or peas, cooked	⅓ cup
Lima beans	½ cup
Peas, green (canned or frozen)	½ cup

Starchy Vegetables

Corn	½ cup
Corn on cob	6" ear
Plantain	½ cup
Potato, baked	1 small (3 ounces)
Potato, mashed	½ cup
Squash, winter (acorn, butternut)	¾ cup
Yam/sweet potato, plain	⅓ cup

Breads

Bagel ½	½ (1 ounce)
Bread sticks	2 (4" long × ½" thick)
Croutons, low-fat	1 cup
English muffin	½
Frankfurter/hamburger bun	½ (1 ounce)
Pita	½ round
Plain roll	1 small (1 ounce)
Raisin bread, unfrosted	1 slice (1 ounce)
Rye/pumpernickel bread	1 slice (1 ounce)
Tortilla	1 (6" round)
White bread (including French or Italian)	1 slice (1 ounce)
Whole wheat bread	1 slice (1 ounce)

Crackers/Snacks, Low-Fat

Animal crackers	8
Graham crackers	3 (1½" squares)
Matzo	3/4 ounces
Melba toast	5 slices
Oyster crackers	24
Popcorn, dry-popped, no fat added	3 cups
Pretzels	3/4 ounce
Rye crisp	4 (2" × 3½")
Saltine-type crackers	6
Whole wheat crackers, no fat added (crisp breads, such as Finn, Kavli, Wasa)	2–4 slices (¼ ounce)

Prepared Starchy Foods

Biscuit (muffinlike, not a cracker/cookie)	1 (2½" diameter)
Chow mein noodles	½ cup
Corn bread	1 (2 ounce, or 2" cube)
Crackers, round butter type	6
French fried potatoes	10 (1½ ounce)
Muffin, plain	1 small
Pancake	2 (4" diameter)
Stuffing, bread (prepared)	¼ cup
Taco shell	2 (6" across)
Waffle	1 (4½" square)
Wheat crackers	4–6 (1 ounce) crackers

— fruit exchanges —
(approximately 15 g carb per serving)

Fresh, Canned, or Pureed

Apple	1 (2" diameter)
Applesauce, unsweetened	1/2 cup
Apricot	4 medium-size
Banana	1/2 (approximately 41/2" long)
Blackberries	3/4 cup
Blueberries	3/4 cup
Cantaloupe	1/3 (5" diameter melon)
Cantaloupe, cubes	1 cup
Cherries	12 large
Cherries, canned	1/2 cup
Figs	2 (2" diameter)
Fruit cocktail, canned	1/2 cup
Grapefruit	1/2 medium-size
Grapefruit, segments	3/4 cup
Grapes	15 small
Honeydew	1/8 (medium-size melon)
Honeydew, cubes	1 cup
Kiwi	1 large
Mandarin oranges	3/4 cup
Mango	1/2 small
Nectarine	1 (11/2" diameter)
Orange	1 (21/2" diameter)
Papaya	1 cup
Peach	1 (23/4" diameter)
Peach, canned	2 halves, or 1/2 cup
Pear	1/2 large or 1 small
Pear, canned	2 halves or 1/2 cup
Persimmon	2 medium-size
Pineapple	3/4 cup
Pineapple, canned	1/3 cup
Plum	2 (2" diameter)
Pomegranate	1/2
Raspberries	1 cup
Strawberries	11/4 cups
Tangerine	2 (21/2" diameter)
Watermelon, cubes	11/4 cups

Fruit: Dried

Apples	4 rings
Apricots	7 halves
Dates	2½ medium-size
Figs	1½
Prunes	3 medium-size
Raisins	2 tablespoons

Fruit Juice

Apple juice/cider	½ cup
Cranberry juice cocktail	⅓ cup
Grapefruit juice	½ cup
Grape juice	⅓ cup
Orange juice	½ cup
Pineapple juice	½ cup
Prune juice	⅓ cup

— milk exchanges —
(approximately 12 g carb per serving)

Skim, ½%, 1%, 2%, or whole milk	1 cup
Low-fat buttermilk	1 cup
Evaporated skim/whole milk	½ cup
Dry nonfat milk	⅓ cup
Plain nonfat, low-fat, or whole-milk yogurt	8 ounces

— vegetable exchanges —
(approximately 5 g carb per serving)

Artichoke	1/2 medium-size
Asparagus	1 cup raw, 1/2 cup cooked
Beans (green, wax, Italian)	1 cup raw, 1/2 cup cooked
Bean sprouts	1 cup raw, 1/2 cup cooked
Beets	1 cup raw, 1/2 cup cooked
Broccoli	1 cup raw, 1/2 cup cooked
Brussels sprouts	1 cup raw, 1/2 cup cooked
Cabbage	1 cup raw, 1/2 cup cooked
Cauliflower	1 cup raw, 1/2 cup cooked
Eggplant	1 cup raw, 1/2 cup cooked
Greens (beet, collard, mustard, turnip)	1 cup raw, 1/2 cup cooked
Kohlrabi	1 cup raw, 1/2 cup cooked
Leeks	1 cup raw, 1/2 cup cooked
Mushrooms	1 cup raw, 1/2 cup cooked
Okra	1 cup raw, 1/2 cup cooked
Onions	1 cup raw, 1/2 cup cooked
Pea pods	1 cup raw, 1/2 cup cooked
Peppers, bell	1 cup raw, 1/2 cup cooked
Rutabaga	1 cup raw, 1/2 cup cooked
Sauerkraut	1 cup raw, 1/2 cup cooked
Spinach	1 cup raw, 1/2 cup cooked
Summer squash (yellow)	1 cup raw, 1/2 cup cooked
Tomato	1 cup raw, 1/2 cup cooked
Tomato/vegetable juice	1/2 cup
Turnips	1 cup raw, 1/2 cup cooked
Water chestnuts	1 cup raw, 1/2 cup cooked
Zucchini	1 cup raw, 1/2 cup cooked

— meat exchanges —
(approximately 0 g carb per serving)

Meats

Beef (steak, ground beef, roast, prime rib, corned beef)	1 ounce
Pork (ham, bacon, chop, cutlet, sparerib, sausage)	1 ounce
Lamb (chop, leg, roast)	1 ounce
Veal (chop, roast, cutlet)	1 ounce
Poultry (chicken, turkey, duck, goose)	1 ounce
Game (venison, rabbit, squirrel, pheasant)	1 ounce
Organ meat (liver, brain, kidney, heart)	1 ounce
Cold cuts (bologna, salami, pimiento loaf)	1 ounce

Seafood

Fish, fresh	1 ounce
Shellfish (shrimp, lobster, crab, clam), fresh	2 ounces
Oysters, fresh	6 medium
Tuna or salmon (canned)	1/4 cup
Sardines (canned)	2 medium-size
Herring (pickled)	1 ounce

Cheese

Cottage cheese	1/2 cup
Grated Parmesan	2 tablespoons
Sliced cheeses (American, blue, Cheddar, Monterey Jack, Swiss)	1 ounce
Diet cheeses	1 ounce
Ricotta	1/4 cup
Mozzarella	1 ounce

Other

Tofu	4 ounces
Peanut butter	1 tablespoon
Egg, whole	1 large
Egg whites	3 whites
Egg substitute	1/4 cup
Hot dog	1

— fat exchanges —
(approximately 0 g carb per serving)

Unsaturated Fats

Avocado	1/8 medium
Margarine	1 teaspoon
Margarine, low-fat	1 tablespoon
Mayonnaise	1 teaspoon
Mayonnaise, reduced-calorie	1 tablespoon
Nuts and seeds:	
Almonds, dry roasted	6 whole
Cashews, dry roasted	1 tablespoon
Pecans	2 whole
Peanuts	20 small or 10 large
Walnuts	2 whole
Other nuts	1 tablespoon
Seeds, pine nuts, sunflower (shelled)	2 tablespoons
Pumpkin seeds	1 teaspoon
Oil (corn, cottonseed, safflower, soybean, sunflower, olive, or peanut)	1 teaspoon
Olives	10 small or 5 large
Salad dressing, mayonnaise-type	2 teaspoons
Salad dressing, mayonnaise-type, reduced-calorie	1 tablespoon
Salad dressing (all varieties)	1 tablespoon
Salad dressing, reduced-calorie	2 tablespoons

Saturated Fats

Butter	1 teaspoon
Bacon	1 slice
Chitterlings	½ ounce
Coconut, shredded	2 tablespoons
Coffee whitener, liquid	2 tablespoons
Coffee whitener, powder	4 teaspoon
Cream, light	2 tablespoons
Cream, sour	2 tablespoons
Cream, heavy (whipping)	1 tablespoon
Cream cheese	1 tablespoon
Salt pork	¼ ounce

tool kit 2

AS I **DESCRIBED** in chapter 3, carb factors represent the percentage of a food's weight that is carbohydrate. Multiply the weight of your prepared food portion (in grams) by the carb factor to calculate the grams of carbohydrate. Only weigh the portion that you plan to consume (without rind, shell, peel, packaging, etc.)

Beans

Baked beans	0.15
Kidney beans	0.16
Lima beans	0.09
Soybeans	0.06

Beverages

Apple juice	0.11
Beer (light)	0.10
Beer (regular)	0.30
Cola beverage	0.10
Cranberry juice	0.14

Daiquiri	0.06
Ginger ale	0.08
Piña colada	0.22
Wine (dry)	0.01
Wine (sweet)	0.11

Breads

Bagel	0.51
Biscuit, plain or buttermilk	0.47
Bread crumbs	0.70
Bread stuffing	0.18
Cornbread	0.45
Croissant	0.43
English muffin	0.33
French bread	0.48
Italian bread	0.47
Raisin bread	0.48
Roll	0.47
Taco shell	0.54
White bread	0.47
Whole wheat bread	0.39

Breakfast Foods

All-Bran	0.43
Apple Jacks	0.87
Cap'n Crunch	0.82
Cheerios	0.67
Cornflakes	0.83
Corn grits	0.12
Cream of wheat	0.11
Frosted Flakes	0.89
Frosted Mini-Wheats	0.71
Froot Loops	0.86
Grape-Nuts	0.72
Lucky Charms	0.79
Oatmeal (prepared)	0.14
Pancakes	0.28

Quaker Oats (dry)	0.61
Raisin Bran	0.63
Rice Krispies	0.85
Shredded Wheat	0.71
Waffle	0.36
Wheaties	0.72

Cakes/Pastries

Angel food cake	0.56
Animal crackers	0.73
Apple pie	0.32
Blueberry muffin	0.45
Blueberry pie	0.33
Boston cream pie	0.41
Chocolate cake (w/frosting)	0.51
Chocolate cake (w/o frosting)	0.51
Chocolate chip cookie	0.60
Chocolate pudding	0.21
Coffeecake	0.44
Cream puff	0.22
Cupcake	0.62
Danish	0.43
Doughnut (glazed)	0.55
Doughnut (plain)	0.48
Éclair, custard-filled, glazed	0.23
Fruitcake	0.57
Graham cracker	0.74
Oatmeal cookie	0.65
Oatmeal-raisin cookie	0.64
Piecrust	0.62
Pound cake	0.48
Pumpkin pie	0.24
Sandwich cookie	0.67
Sponge cake	0.60

Condiments/Spreads/Sauces

Catsup	0.25
Croutons	0.68
Gravy (beef)	0.04
Hummus	0.08
Maple syrup	0.67
Peanut butter, smooth	0.13
Salad dressing, Italian	0.10
Tomato paste	0.15
Tomato sauce	0.07

Dairy

Cheddar cheese	0.01
Cream cheese	0.02
Egg	0.01
Frozen yogurt	0.22
Ice cream, chocolate	0.27
Ice cream, vanilla	0.23
Ice cream, vanilla soft-serve	0.22
Milk	0.05
Mozzarella cheese	0.02
Parmesan cheese	0.03
Ricotta cheese	0.05
Sour cream	0.04
Swiss cheese	0.03

Fruit (fresh unless otherwise indicated)

Apple	0.12
Applesauce, sweetened	0.18
Applesauce, unsweetened	0.10
Apricot	0.08
Banana	0.21
Blackberries	0.07
Blueberries	0.11
Cantaloupe	0.07
Cherries	0.14

Cranberries	0.08
Grapefruit	0.06
Grapes	0.16
Honeydew	0.08
Kiwifruit	0.11
Mango	0.15
Orange	0.09
Orange (with peel)	0.11
Peach	0.09
Pear	0.12
Pineapple	0.11
Plum	0.11
Raisins	0.75
Raspberries	0.04
Strawberries	0.04
Tangerine	0.08
Watermelon	0.06

Grains/Pasta

Couscous, cooked	0.21
Egg noodles	0.23
Macaroni and cheese	0.10
Macaroni, cooked	0.27
Rice noodles, cooked	0.23
Rice, brown	0.21
Rice, white	0.27
Spaghetti, cooked	0.26

Mixed/Combination Foods

Beef stew	0.05
Chicken pot pie	0.18
Chili with beans	0.07
Coleslaw	0.10
Onion rings	0.36
Pizza, pepperoni	0.27
Pizza, plain	0.32

Potato salad	0.09
Shrimp, breaded and fried	0.11
Tuna salad	0.09

Snacks

Almonds	0.07
Almonds, honey roasted	0.14
Beef jerky	0.09
Cashews	0.29
Cheese crackers	0.55
Matzo	0.80
Peanuts, dry-roasted	0.13
Pecans	0.04
Pistachios	0.17
Popcorn, air-popped	0.62
Popcorn, caramel-coated	0.73
Popcorn, cheese-flavored	0.41
Popcorn, oil-popped	0.47
Potato chips	0.48
Pretzels	0.76
Saltine crackers	0.68
Spanish peanuts	0.08
Tortilla chips	0.57
Walnuts	0.07

Candies

Baking chocolate (bittersweet)	0.64
Butterscotch candy	0.95
Caramel	0.75
Fudge	0.78
Hard candy	0.98
Jellybeans	0.93
M&M's (plain)	0.68
Milk chocolate	0.55
Milk chocolate–coated peanuts	0.44
Milk chocolate–coated raisins	0.64
Rice Krispies Treats	0.79

Semisweet chocolate	0.57
Sherbet	0.30

Vegetables

Artichoke	0.02
Artichokes	0.05
Asparagus, raw	0.02
Broccoli, raw	0.02
Cabbage, raw	0.03
Carrots, raw	0.06
Cauliflower	0.02
Celery	0.01
Corn	0.16
Cucumbers	0.01
Green beans	0.02
Lettuce	0.01
Mushrooms, raw	0.02
Onions, raw	0.06
Peas, raw	0.09
Peppers, bell, raw	0.04
Pickles	0.02
Potato pancakes	0.26
Potato, baked	0.22
Potatoes, French fried	0.27
Potatoes, hash brown	0.26
Potatoes, mashed	0.15
Potatoes, scalloped	0.08
Spinach, cooked	0.01
Squash, summer	0.02
Squash, winter	0.10
Sweet potato	0.21
Tomato, raw	0.03
Yam	0.23

tool kit 3

GLYCEMIC INDEX VALUES

AS DESCRIBED IN chapter 4, the glycemic index refers to the *speed* with which various foods convert into sugar (glucose) in the bloodstream. Higher-numbered foods tend to digest and convert to glucose very quickly; lower-numbered foods convert more slowly. Pure glucose is given a score of 100. For a more detailed glycemic index list, visit www.glycemicindex.com, or look for the current annual edition of *The New Glucose Revolution Shopper's Guide to GI Values* at your favorite local or online bookseller.

Baby Foods

Apple, apricot, banana cereal	56
Chicken and noodle with vegetables, strained	67
Formula	36
Porridge	59
Rice cereal	95
Rice pudding	59
Corn and rice	65

Bakery Products

Angel food cake	67
Banana muffin	65
Blueberry muffin	59
Bran muffin	60
Chocolate cake, made from mix with chocolate frosting	38
Corn muffin	102
Croissant	67
Crumpet	69
Cupcake, iced	73
Doughnut, cake type	76
Flan cake	65
Oatmeal	69
Pancakes	67
Pancakes, buckwheat, gluten-free	102
Pound cake	54
Scones	92
Sponge cake	46
Vanilla cake, made from mix with vanilla frosting	42
Waffles	76

Beverages, Mixes, and Sport Drinks

AllSport (orange)	53
Coca-Cola	63
Cytomax (orange)	62
Fanta orange soda	68
Gatorade (orange)	89
GatorLode (orange)	100
Malted milk powder	45
Nestlé Quik (Nesquik) (chocolate, dissolved in milk)	41
Nestlé Quik (Nesquik) (chocolate, dissolved in water)	53
Powerade (orange)	65
Smoothie, raspberry	33

Breads

100% whole-grain bread	62
Bagel, frozen	72
Baguette, plain	95
Barley bread	67
Bread stuffing	74
Buckwheat bread	47
Gluten-free white bread	80
Hamburger bun	61
Italian bread	73
Kaiser rolls	73
Melba toast	70
Middle Eastern flatbread	97
Oat bran bread	44
Pita bread	57
Rye bread	58
Whole wheat bread	70
White bread	73

Breakfast Foods

All-Bran	42
Multi-Bran Chex	58
Bran Flakes	74
Cheerios	74
Corn Chex	83
Corn Pops	80
Cornflakes	81
Cream of Wheat	66
Crispix	87
Froot Loops	69
Golden Grahams	71
Grapenuts	75
Honey Smacks	71
Life	66
Mini-Wheats	58
Oatmeal (rolled oats)	58
Oatmeal (quick oats)	65
Muesli	66
Pop-Tarts	70

Puffed wheat	74
Raisin Bran	61
Rice Krispies	82
Shredded Wheat	75
Special K	69
Total	76

Cereal Grains

Amaranth	97
Barley, pearled	25
Buckwheat	54
Cornmeal	69
Couscous	65
Millet	71
Rice, long-grain white	56
Rice, white	64
Rice, basmati, white	58
Rice, brown	55
Rice, glutinous	98
Rice, instant, white	69
Rice, jasmine	109
Rye, whole kernels	34
Sweet corn	53
Taco shells	68
Wheat, cracked (bulgur)	48
Wheat, whole kernels	41

Dairy and Dairy Alternatives

Custard	43
Ice cream, high fat/premium	38
Ice cream, low fat	50
Ice cream, regular	61
Milk (whole)	40
Milk (skim)	32
Milk, condensed, sweetened	61
Pudding, instant	44
Soy milk	44

Soy smoothie	30
Soy yogurt	50
Yogurt, low fat	33
Yogurt, low fat, sweetened w/aspartame	14
Yogurt, nonfat, sweetened w/Splenda and acesulfame-K	24

Fruit

Apple	38
Apricot, fresh	57
Apricot, canned in light syrup	64
Banana	52
Cantaloupe	65
Cherries	22
Dates	103
Figs	61
Fruit cocktail, canned	55
Grapefruit	25
Grapes	46
Kiwi	53
Lychees, canned in syrup	79
Mango	51
Marmalade, orange	48
Orange	42
Papaya	59
Peach, fresh	42
Peach, canned in heavy syrup	58
Peach, canned in natural juice	38
Peach, canned in light syrup	52
Pear, fresh	38
Pear, canned in pear juice	44
Pineapple	46
Plum	39
Prunes	29
Raisins	64
Strawberries	40
Strawberry jam	51
Sultanas (golden raisins)	56
Watermelon	72

Juices

Apple juice, unsweetened	40
Blueberry juice	58
Carrot juice	43
Cranberry juice cocktail	68
Grape juice	58
Grapefruit juice	48
Orange juice	52
Pineapple juice, unsweetened	46
Pomegranate juice	67
Tomato juice	38

Legumes

Baked beans	48
Black-eyed beans	42
Butter beans	31
Chickpeas (garbanzo beans)	28
Kidney beans	28
Lentils	29
Marrowfat peas	39
Navy beans	38
Pinto beans	39
Romano beans	46
Soybeans	18

Meal Replacements and Energy Bars

Boost High Protein (vanilla) meal	59
Burn-it bar (chocolate)	29
Burn-it bar (peanut butter)	23
Fibre Plus bar	78
Ironman PR Bar	39
Just Right bar	72
LEAN Nutribar	31
MetRx bar (vanilla)	74
Nutrimeal drink powder	26
Power bar (chocolate)	56
Pure-protein bar (chocolate chip)	30

Pure-protein bar (peanut butter)	22
Pure-protein bar (strawberry shortcake)	43
Strawberry Crunch bar	77
Sustain bar	57
Ultra Pure Protein Shake (cappuccino)	47
Ultra Pure Protein Shake (chocolate)	37
Ultra Pure Protein Shake (strawberry shortcake)	42
Ultra Pure Protein Shake (vanilla ice cream)	32

Mixed Meals/Convenience Foods

Chicken nuggets (breaded)	46
Fish sticks	38
Lean Cuisine chicken and rice	36
Peanut butter sandwich	59
Pizza (cheese)	60
Pizza (supreme, pan)	36
Pizza (vegetarian, thin crust)	49
Sausage	28
Spaghetti Bolognese	52
Sushi	52

Nutritional Supplements

ChoiceDM (vanilla)	23
Enercal Plus	61
Ensure	50
Ensure pudding	36
Glucerna (vanilla)	31
Resource Diabetic (French vanilla)	34
Sustagen with extra fiber	33
Sustagen instant pudding	27
Ultracal with fiber	40

Pasta and Noodles

Capellini	45
Fettuccine	40
Gnocchi	68
Linguine, thick	46
Linguine, thin	52
Macaroni	45
Macaroni and cheese, boxed	64
Noodles, instant	47
Ravioli, meat-filled	39
Rice pasta	92
Rice vermicelli	58
Spaghetti, boiled 20 minutes	61
Spaghetti, boiled 5 minutes	38
Tortellini, cheese	50
Vermicelli	35

Snack Foods

Arrowroot cookies	65
Cashews	22
Chocolate (milk chocolate)	43
Corn chips	63
Crackers, plain	74
Fruit Roll-Ups	99
Graham wafers	74
Jelly beans	78
Kudos bar (chocolate chip)	62
Life Saver (peppermint)	70
M&M's peanut	33
Mars Bar	68
Nutella spread	33
Peanuts	14
Popcorn, microwave	72
Potato chips	54
Pretzels	83
Rice cakes	82
Rye crispbread	63
Shortbread	64
Skittles	70

Snickers bar	55
Stoned Wheat Thins	67
Twix cookie bar	44
Vanilla wafers	77

Soups

Black bean	64
Green pea	66
Lentil	44
Minestrone	39
Split pea	60
Tomato	38

Sugars and Sweeteners

Fructose	19
Glucose	100
Honey	55
Lactitol	2
Lactose	46
Sucrose	68
Xylitol	8

Vegetables

Beets	64
Carrots	47
Cassava	46
Corn	54
Parsnips	97
Peas, green	48
Potato, baked	85
Potato, French fried	75
Potato, fresh, mashed	74
Potato, instant mashed	85
Pumpkin	75
Rutabaga	72

Sweet potato	61
Tapioca	81
Taro	55
Yam	37

tool kit 4

C = Total Carbohydrate (grams)

F = Fiber (grams)

When blank, fiber grams are unknown

Eating "In"

Dairy

	C	F
Butter, 1 tbsp	0	0
Buttermilk, low fat, 1 cup	12	0
Cheese fondue, 1 cup	8	0
Cheese product, Kraft Singles, 1 slice	2	0
Cheese product, Velveeta Light, 1 oz	3	0
Cheese product, Velveeta Spread, 1 oz	3	0
Cheese sauce, ¼ cup	3	0
Cheese spread, cream cheese base, 2 tbsp	1	0
Cheese, blue, 1 oz	1	0
Cheese, brick, 1 oz	0	0
Cheese, brie, 1 oz	0	0
Cheese, camembert, 1 oz	0	0
Cheese, caraway, 1 oz	0	0
Cheese, cheddar, 1 oz	0	0
Cheese, cheshire, 1 oz	1	0
Cheese, colby, 1 oz	0	0
Cheese, edam, 1 oz	0	0
Cheese, feta, ¼ cup, crumbled	1	0
Cheese, fontina, 1 oz	0	0
Cheese, goat, 1 oz	1	0
Cheese, gouda, 1 oz	1	0
Cheese, limburger, 1 oz	0	0
Cheese, monterey, 1 oz	0	0
Cheese, mozzarella, part skim milk, 1 oz	1	0
Cheese, muenster, 1 oz	0	0
Cheese, neufchatel, 1 oz	1	0
Cheese, parmesan, 1 oz	1	0
Cheese, parmesan, shredded/grated, 1 tbsp	0	0
Cheese, pasteurized process, american, 1 slice	1	0
Cheese, provolone, 1 oz	0	0
Cheese, ricotta, part skim milk, ½ cup	6	0
Cheese, romano, 1 oz	1	0
Cheese, roquefort, 1 oz	1	0

	C	F
Cheese, swiss, 1 oz	1	0
Cheez Whiz cheese sauce, 2 tbsp	3	0
Cheez Whiz Light cheese product, 2 tbsp	6	0
Chocolate milk, 1 cup	36	1
Chocolate milk, low fat, 1 cup	26	1
Chocolate milk, reduced fat, 1 cup	30	2
Cottage cheese, creamed, large or small curd, ½ cup	3	0
Cottage cheese, fat free, ½ cup	3	0
Cottage cheese, low fat, ½ cup	3	0
Cream cheese, 2 tbsp	1	0
Cream cheese, low fat, 2 tbsp	2	0
Cream substitute, 1 container	2	0
Cream topping: Cool Whip, 2 tbsp	2	0
Cream topping: Reddi-Wip original, 1 tbsp	1	0
Cream, fluid, half and half, 1 oz	1	0
Cream, fluid, light (coffee cream or table cream), 1 oz	1	0
Cream, fluid, light whipping, 1 cup	1	0
Cream, half and half, fat free, 1 oz	3	0
Cream, sour, cultured, 1 tbsp	0	0
Cream, sour, reduced fat, cultured, 1 tbsp	0	0
Custard, ½ cup	19	0
Egg substitute, liquid, ½ cup	1	0
Egg, whole, cooked, fried, 1 large	0	0
Egg, whole, cooked, hard-boiled, ½ cup, chopped	1	0
Egg, whole, cooked, scrambled, ½ cup	2	0
Eggnog, 1 cup	34	0
Flan, caramel custard, dry mix, 1 package	78	0
Flan, caramel custard, prepared, ½ cup	26	0
Frozen yogurt, nonfat, ½ cup	30	0

	C	F
Frozen fruit bar, no sugar added, 1 bar	3	0
Frozen yogurt, low fat, ½ cup	28	0
Half & half, 1 tbsp	1	0
Half & half, fat free, 2 tbsp	3	0
Ice cream, chocolate, ½ cup	16	1
Ice cream, chocolate or caramel covered, with nuts, 1 bar	17	0
Ice cream, chocolate, "light," ½ cup	20	1
Ice cream, chocolate, light, no sugar added, ½ cup	18	1
Ice cream, strawberry, ½ cup	16	1
Ice cream, vanilla, ½ cup	17	1
Ice cream, vanilla, light, ½ cup	20	0
Ice cream, vanilla, soft-serve, ½ cup	19	1
Ice cream, vanilla, no sugar added, ½ cup	15	0
Margarine, 1 tbsp	0	0
Milk (1%), 1 cup	12	0
Milk (buffalo), 1 cup	13	0
Milk (fat free or skim), 1 cup	12	0
Milk (goat), 1 cup	11	0
Milk (human), 1 cup	17	0
Milk (reduced fat/2%), 1 cup	11	0
Milk (sheep), 1 cup	13	0
Milk (soy), 1 cup	12	3
Milk, chocolate beverage, hot cocoa, homemade, 1 cup	27	3
Sour cream, fat free, 2 tbsp	6	0
Sour cream, fat free, Breakstone's, 2 tbsp	5	0
Sour cream, imitation, cultured, 1 cup	15	0
Sour cream, light, 2 tbsp	2	0
Sour cream, reduced fat, Breakstone's, 2 tbsp	2	0
Tapioca, ½ cup	15	0
Yogurt, Breyers Lowfat Strawberry, 8 oz	41	0
Yogurt, Breyers Smooth & Creamy Lowfat Strawberry, 8 oz	45	1
Yogurt, fruit variety, nonfat, 1 cup	47	0

	C	F
Yogurt, fruit, low fat, average, 8 oz	45	0
Yogurt, fruit, low fat, with low calorie sweetener, 1 8 oz container	42	0
Yogurt, plain, low fat, 1 cup	17	0
Yogurt, plain, skim milk, 1 cup	19	0
Yogurt, plain, whole milk, 8 oz	11	0

FRUIT

	C	F
Apple, medium, 2¾" diam or 6 oz	21	4
Apple Juice, 8 oz	30	0
Apple large, 3¼" diam or 8 oz	32	6
Apple, raw, without skin, 1 cup	14	1
Apple, small, 2¼" diam or 4 oz	17	3
Apricot, whole, medium	6	1
Apricots, dried, ½ cup	40	4
Banana (6–7 inches), small	24	2
Banana (less than 6 inches), extra small	19	2
Banana (7–8 inches), medium	28	3
Banana (8–9 inches), large	32	3
Banana (greater than 9 inches), extra large	36	4
Banana, mashed, 1 cup	48	4
Blackberries, raw, ½ cup	7	4
Blueberries, raw, ½ cup	10	1
Cantaloupe, raw, 1 cup	14	2
Carambola, (starfruit), raw, ½ cup	5	2
Casaba, raw, 1 cup	11	1
Chayote, fruit, raw 5¾ inch diameter, ½ cup	4	0
Cherimoya, raw peeled and seedless, 1 fruit	55	7
Cherry, Maraschino, 1	2	0
Cherries, sweet, raw, 1 cup	19	2
Clementines, raw, 1 fruit	9	1
Coconut, dried/sweetened, ½ cup	22	2
Coconut, shredded, ½ cup	6	1
Cranberries, raw, ½ cup	6	2

	C	F
Cranberry Juice Cocktail, 8 oz	36	0
Currants, red and white, raw, 1 cup	15	5
Currants, zante, dried, 1 cup	107	10
Dates, medjool, 1 date	18	2
Elderberries, raw, ½ cup	13	5
Figs, raw, 1 large	12	2
Fruit butter, apple, 1 tablespoon	8	0
Fruit Cocktail in heavy syrup, 1 cup	53	3
Fruit Cocktail in light syrup, 1 cup	32	4
Fruit Salad, mixed melons, berries, 1 cup	20	3
Gooseberries, raw, 1 cup	15	6
Grape Juice, 8 oz	40	0
Grapefruit, half of medium	10	1
Grapefruit, half of small	8	1
Grapefruit, raw, pieces, 1 cup	19	3
Grapefruit, half of large	13	2
Grapes, red or green, 1 grape	1	0
Grapes, red or green, 1 cup	29	1
Guavas, common, raw, 1 cup	24	9
Guavas, strawberry, raw, 1 cup	42	13
Honeydew, raw, 1 cup	16	1
Jackfruit, raw, ½ cup	25	4
Kiwi fruit, fresh, raw, ½ cup	13	2
Kumquats, raw, 2 fruit	3	1
Lemon Juice, 1 tbsp	1	0
Lemons, raw, without peel, 1 fruit aprox 2" diam	5	2
Lemons, raw, without peel, ½ cup	10	3
Limes, raw, 1 fruit	7	2
Litchis, raw, ½ cup	15	1
Loganberries, frozen, 1 cup	19	7
Mulberries, raw, 1 cup	14	2
Nectarines, raw, 1 medium	12	2
Orange, small	11	2
Orange, medium	15	3
Orange, large	21	4
Orange Juice, 8 oz	26	0
Oranges, raw, without rind, 1 cup	21	4
Papaya, 1 small	15	3

	C	F
Papaya, raw, 1 cup	14	3
Papaya/Peach Nectar, 8 oz	31	0
Passion Fruit Juice, 8 oz	35	0
Passion-fruit, (granadilla), raw, ½ cup	27	12
Peach, medium	14	3
Peach halves, raw, 1 cup	16	3
Pear Nectar, 8 oz	40	0
Pear, whole, medium	24	4
Pears, raw, 1 cup	26	5
Persimmons, Japanese, raw, 1 fruit	31	6
Pineapple Juice, 8 oz	35	0
Pineapple, raw, ½ cup	10	1
Plantains, raw, 1 cup	47	3
Plum, raw, medium	10	2
Plum, raw, large	15	3
Plum, raw, small	7	1
Pomegranates, raw, ½ fruit	15	2
Prickly pears, raw, 1 cup	14	5
Prune (dried plum), small	4	0
Prune (dried plum), medium	5	1
Prune (dried plum), large	6	1
Prune Juice, 8 oz	45	2
Quinces, raw, 3 fruit	14	2
Raisins, seedless, 2 tbsp (1 oz)	22	2
Raspberries, raw, ½ cup	7	4
Strawberries, raw, ½ cup (3 medium)	6	2
Strawberry/Raspberry Juice, 8 oz	23	0
Tangerine Juice, 8 oz	25	0
Watermelon, raw, 1 cup	12	1

MEAT

	C	F
Bacon, 2 strips	0	0
Bacon Bits, 1 tsp	4	0
Bacon, Canadian-style, 2 slices	1	0
Bacon, turkey, 1 cup, pieces	3	0
Barbecue beef, 4 oz	8	0

	C	F
Bass, 4 oz	0	0
Beef, cured, 3 oz	1	0
Beef, ground, 1 patty	0	0
Beef, loin, 3 oz	0	0
Beef, rib, 3 oz	0	0
Beef, round, 3 oz	0	0
Bologna, 1 slice	1	0
Bologna, chicken or turkey, 1 slice	2	0
Bologna, low fat, 1 slice	2	0
Brain, cooked, simmered, 3 oz	3	0
Calamari, breaded/fried, 1 cup	10	0
Catfish, baked, 4 oz	0	0
Catfish, breaded/fried, 1 fillet	7	0
Caviar, black and red, granular, 1 tbsp	1	0
Chicken breast, baked, with or without skin, 1 breast	0	0
Chicken breast, battered & fried, 1 breast	12	0
Chicken breast, flour coated, 1 breast	7	0
Chicken drumstick, baked or roasted, with or without skin, 1 drumstick	0	0
Chicken drumstick, battered & fried, 1 drumstick	7	0
Chicken drumstick, flour coated, 1 drumstick	1	0
Chicken liver, 4 oz	3	0
Chicken nuggets, 5	16	0
Chicken thigh, baked or roasted, with or without skin, 1 thigh	0	0
Chicken thigh, battered & fried, 1 thigh	8	0
Chicken thigh, flour coated, 1 thigh	2	0
Chicken wing, baked or roasted, with or without skin, 1 wing	0	0
Chicken wing, battered & fried, 1 wing	5	0
Chicken wing, flour coated, 1 wing	1	0
Chili with Beans, 1 cup	29	11
Chorizo, pork and beef, 1 link	1	0

	C	F
Clams, breaded/fried, ¾ cup	39	0
Clams, raw, 4 large/9 small	2	0
Cod, 4 oz	0	0
Corned Beef Hash, 1 cup	29	6
Crab Cake, 1 medium	16	0
Crab, cooked or steamed, 3 oz	0	0
Crab, imitation stix, made from surimi, 3 oz	9	0
Fish fillet, battered or breaded, and fried, 1 fillet	8	0
Fish sticks, breaded & fried, 1 stick	3	0
Frankfurter, beef, 1 frankfurter	2	0
Frankfurter, beef and pork, 1 frankfurter	1	0
Frankfurter, beef and pork, low fat, 1 cup, sliced	7	0
Frankfurter, chicken, 1 frankfurter	3	0
Gefilte fish, sweet recipe, 1 piece	3	0
Gravy (beef, chicken, turkey, or mushroom), ¼ cup	3	0
Gravy, au jus, ¼ cup	2	0
Ham, sliced, extra lean, 3 slices	2	0
Herring, pickled, ½ cup	6	0
Kielbasa, Polish, 1 2 oz link	1	0
Knockwurst, pork & beef, 1 link	2	0
Lamb, 3 oz	0	0
Liver, 3 oz	4	0
Liver, cooked, pan-fried, 3 oz	4	0
Lobster tail, cooked, 1 medium	1	0
Lobster, cooked, 1 cup	2	0
Lobster, cooked, 1 cup	2	0
Meatball, Swedish, 1 medium	1	0
Octopus, cooked, 3 oz	4	0
Olive loaf, pork, 1 slice	3	0
Oysters, breaded/fried, 6 medium	10	0
Oysters, raw, 6 medium	3	0
Pork, 3 oz	0	0
Salami, 1 oz	1	0
Salmon cake, 1 patty	7	0
Salmon steak, 8 oz	0	0
Salmon, smoked, ½ cup	0	0

	C	F
Sardines, 2 medium	0	0
Sausage, beef, medium	0	0
Sausage, Italian, 1 link	3	0
Sausage, patty or link, 1 piece	1	0
Sausage, pork, 1 sausage	4	0
Scallops, breaded/fried, 6 medium	38	0
Scallops, broiled, 6 medium	2	0
Scrapple, pork, 1 link	0	0
Shark, 4 oz	0	0
Shrimp cocktail, 1 medium	1	0
Shrimp, breaded and fried, 1 medium	1	0
Shrimp, breaded and fried, 1 large	3	0
Shrimp, popcorn, each	1	0
SPAM Luncheon Meat, 1 serving	2	0
Surimi (imitation crab), 4 oz	7	0
Swordfish, 4 oz	0	0
Tofu, 4 oz	3	0
Trout, 4 oz	0	0
Tuna, 4 oz	0	0
Turkey and gravy, frozen, 1 cup	11	0
Turkey, roasted, 4 oz	0	0
Veal, breaded/fried, 3 oz	9	0
Veal, not breaded, 3 oz	0	0

POURABLES

SOUPS

	C	F
Beef Consomme, 1 cup	2	0
Bouillabaisse, 1 cup	10	0
Boullion Cube, 1 cube	1	0
Chicken & Rice, 1 cup	9	0
Chicken Consomme, 1 cup	2	0
Chicken Jambalaya, 1 cup	8	0
Chicken Noodle, 1 cup	12	0
Clam Chowder, 1 cup	17	0
Corn Chowder, 1 cup	16	0
Cream of Broccoli, 1 cup	20	0

	C	F
Cream of Potato, 1 cup	25	0
Cream of Mushroom, 1 cup	20	0
French Onion, 1 cup	25	0
Gazpacho, 1 cup	13	0
Lentil, 1 cup	28	10
Lobster Bisque, 1 cup	10	0
Matzo Ball (w/1 ball), 1 cup	24	0
Mulligatawny, 1 cup	8	0
Split Pea, 1 cup	18	8
Vegetable, 1 cup	18	3
Vichysoisse, 1 cup	15	0
Tomato, 1 cup	20	1
Tomato Bisque, 1 cup	23	1

DIPS, SAUCES, & SPREADS

	C	F
Barbecue Sauce, 1 tbsp	6	0
Bearnaise Sauce, ¼ cup	5	0
Buffalo Wing Sauce, 1 tbsp	2	0
Cocktail Sauce, ¼ cup	15	0
Cooking Spray, 3-second spray	0	0
Cranberry Sauce, ¼ cup	27	1
Gravy, beef, chicken, or turkey, average, ¼ cup	3	0
Guacamole, 2 tbsp	2	0
Honey Mustard Dip, 2 tbsp	10	0
Horseradish, 1 tsp	0	0
Hummus, 2 tbsp	5	1
Jalapeno Dip, 2 tbsp	3	0
Ketchup, 1 tbsp	4	0
Miso Paste, 1 tbsp	5	0
Mushroom Sauce, ½ cup	5	0
Mustard, 1 tbsp	1	0
Nacho Cheese, 2 tbsp	3	0
Pesto, ¼ cup	2	0
Relish, 1 tbsp	5	0
Salsa, average, 2 tbsp	3	1
Sauerkraut, ½ cup	5	3
Sour Cream & Onion Dip, 2 tbsp	0	0
Soy Sauce, 1 tbsp	0	0

	C	F
Spaghetti Sauce, extra thick, ½ cup	19	2
Spaghetti Sauce, reg, average, ½ cup	11	1
Steak Sauce, average, 1 tbsp	3	0
Sweet & Sour Sauce, 2 tbsp	10	0
Tabasco Sauce, 1 tsp	0	0
Teriyaki Sauce, 1 tbsp	3	0
Tomato Sauce, average, ½ cup	9	0
Tzatziki, 2 tbsp	1	0
Vegetable Oil, 1 tbsp	0	0
Vinegar, white or red, ⅛ cup	1	0
Wocesteshire Sauce, 1 tsp	1	0

DRESSINGS

	C	F
Balsamic Vinaigrette, 2 tbsp	4	0
Balsamic Vinaigrette, fat free, 2 tbsp	1	0
Balsamic Vinaigrette, light, 2 tbsp	2	0
Blue Cheese, 2 tbsp	2	0
Blue Cheese, Light, 2 tbsp	1	0
Caesar, 2 tbsp	2	0
Caesar, light, 2 tbsp	1	0
French, 2 tbsp	5	0
French, fat free, 2 tbsp	4	0
French, light, 2 tbsp	2	0
Italian, 2 tbsp	5	0
Italian, fat free, 2 tbsp	4	0
Italian, light, 2 tbsp	2	0
Ranch, 2 tbsp	3	0
Ranch, fat free, 2 tbsp	2	0
Ranch, light, 2 tbsp	3	0
Thousand Island, 2 tbsp	5	0
Thousand Island, fat free, 2 tbsp	3	0
Thousand Island, light, 2 tbsp	3	0

BEVERAGES

	C	F
Beer, nonalcoholic, average, 12-oz bottle/can	14	0
Boost energy drink, 1 cup	41	0
Café Mocha, 1 cup	15	0
Caffe Latte, average, 1 cup	8	0
Cappuccino, average, 1 cup	6	0
Chocolate drink, average, 1 cup	30	0

	C	F
Club Soda, 1 cup	0	0
Coffee, brewed w/1 packet sugar, 1 cup	7	0
Coffee, brewed, black or w/cream, 1 cup	1	0
Coffee, brewed, w/milk, 1 cup	2	0
Cola, diet, 1 cup	0	0
Cola, regular, 1 cup	25	0
Cola, regular, 12-oz can	37	0
Cream Soda, 1 cup	42	0
Ensure nutritional supplement, 1 cup	40	0
Espresso, regular, single serving	1	0
Frappuccino, 1½ cups	39	0
Gatorade, 1 cup	14	0
Ginger Ale, 1 cup	20	0
Hot Chocolate w/milk, 1 cup	25	0
Hot Cocoa w/milk, 1 cup	22	0
Iced Tea, sugar-sweetened, 1 cup	25	0
Iced Tea, unsweetened, 1 cup	0	0
Kool Aid, average, 1 cup	17	0
Lemon Lime Soda, 1 cup	38	0
Lemonade, average, 1 cup	20	0
Orange Soda, 1 cup	30	0
Powerade, 1 cup	16	0
Red Bull, 1 cup	27	0
Root Beer, 1 cup	28	0
Seltzer, 1 cup	0	0
Soy beverage, average, 1 cup	22	0
Tea, brewed, 1 cup	0	0
Tea, herbal, 1 cup	0	0
Tonic Water, 1 cup	22	0

ALCOHOLIC BEVERAGES

	C	F
Alabama Slammer, 1 shooter	2	0
Amaretto Sours, 1 shooter	19	0
Bacardi, 12 oz	33	0
Bahama Mama, 4 oz	16	0
Beer, light, average, 12-oz bottle/can	5	0
Beer, regular, average, 12-oz bottle/can	11	0
Bloody Mary, 1 average	16	0

	C	F
Blue Lady, 1 average	16	0
Blushin' Russian, 1 average	47	0
Brandy Alexander, 1 average	17	0
Champagne, average, ½ cup	2	0
Cherry Blossom, 1 average	5	0
Cider, dry, 1 cup	8	0
Cider, sweet, 1 cup	10	0
Cosmopolitan, 1 average	12	0
Cranium Meltdown, 1 shooter	2	0
Daiquiri, 1 average	4	0
Daiquiri, frozen, w/fruit, 1 average	10	1
Fuzzy Navel, 1 shooter	7	0
Gin & Tonic, 1 average	22	0
Grasshopper, 1 average	30	0
Hard Lemonade, average, 12-oz bottle/can	34	0
Harvey Wallbanger, 1 average	17	0
Highball, 1 average	3	0
Hurricane, 4 oz	16	0
Irish Coffee, 1 cup	6	0
Kahlua & Cream, 1 average	10	0
Kamakazie, 1 shooter	2	0
Kook-Aid, 1 shooter	14	0
L.A. Sunrise, 1 average	21	0
Lady Killer, 1 average	20	0
Liqueur Coffee, average, 1 cup	16	0
London Rock, 1 average	10	0
Long Island Iced Tea w/diet cola, 1 average	6	0
Long Island Iced Tea, w/cola, 1 average	31	0
Mai Tai, 1 average	16	0
Manhattan, 1 average	3	0
Margarita, 1 average	14	0
Martini, 1 average	0	0
Mint Julep, 1 average	4	0
Mojito, 1 average	6	0
Mud Slide, 1 shooter	17	0
Pina Colada, 1 average	40	0
Pineapple Bomber, 1 shooter	13	0
Rainbow Room, 1 average	14	0

	C	F
Screwdriver, 1 average	14	0
Sex on the Beach, 1 average	26	0
Singapore Sling, 1 average	9	0
Spirits/Liquors, 1 shot	0	0
Spritzer w/wine, 1 average	2	0
Tequila Sunrise, 1 average	25	0
Tom & Jerry, 1 average	8	0
Tom Collins, 1 average	12	0
Turbo, 1 shooter	3	0
Whiskey Sour, 1 average	5	0
White Russian, 1 average	16	0
Wine Cooler, average, 12 oz	35	0
Wine, table, average, ½ cup	3	0

SNACKS

SALTY/CRUNCHY SNACKS

	C	F
Almonds, ½ cup	16	6
Banana chips, ½ cup	21	3
Cashews, ½ cup (8 med)	23	2
Cheese Crackers, bite-size, 27	16	1
Cheese puffs and curls, 1 cup	15	0
Cheese puffs and twists, low fat, 1 cup	17	0
Chex Mix, ½ cup	17	2
Corn Chips, small bag, small (1oz) bag	15	1
Corn Puffs, 1 cup	12	0
Cracker sandwich, cheese or peanut butter, 6-pack	23	1
Crackers, saltines (includes oyster, soda, soup), 1 cup, crushed	50	2
Jerky (beef), 1 oz stick	3	0
Macadamia nuts, ½ cup	8	4
Melba toast, 1 cracker	11	1
Peanuts, honey roasted, ½ cup	25	6
Peanuts, roasted, ½ cup	12	6
Peanut Butter, 2 tbsp	7	2
Peanut Butter, reduced fat, 2 tbsp	14	2
Pecans, ½ cup	12	5
Pistachios, ¼ cup	7	3

	C	F
Popcorn, air popped, 1 cup	4	1
Popcorn, caramel coated, 1 cup	15	1
Popcorn, cheese flavored, 1 cup	4	1
Popcorn, microwave, average bag, 12 cups	50	12
Popcorn, microwave, kettle/sweet, average bag, 12 cups	46	9
Popcorn, microwave, light, average bag, 12 cups	54	15
Popcorn, microwave, mini bag, 6 cups	24	6
Popcorn, movie theater, with or without butter, small (6 cups)	30	6
Popcorn, movie theater, with or without butter, medium (14 cups)	70	14
Popcorn, movie theater, with or without butter, large (20 cups)	100	20
Popcorn, oil popped, 1 cup	5	1
Popcorn, small box, 2 oz	28	5
Pork rinds, ⅔ cup	1	0
Potato chips made with olestra, small bag, approx 17 chips	17	1
Potato chips, baked, small bag, approx 17 chips	24	2
Potato chips, reduced fat, small bag, approx 17 chips	18	1
Potato chips, small bag, approx 17 chips	16	1
Potato crisps (stackable, in can), 14 chips	15	1
Potato crisps (stackable, in can), low fat, 14 chips	20	1
Potato sticks, ½ cup	10	1
Pretzel (soft), bites, 5	29	1
Pretzel (soft), large twist, each	83	2
Pretzel (soft), regular twist, each	41	1
Pretzel nuggets, small, each	2	0
Pretzel rod, each	9	0
Pretzel Sticks, thin, 20	20	1
Pretzel twist, "Hard/Sourdough," each	22	1
Pretzel twists, Specials/Old-Tyme, each	8	0
Pretzel twists, standard, each	3	0
Pretzel twists, thin, each	2	0
Pretzels, chocolate covered, 3 mini	23	0

	C	F
Pretzels, chocolate covered, 1 regular	20	0
Pretzels, mini, 20	25	1
Pretzels, pennysticks, braided twists or logs, each	3	0
Rice cake, average, 1 cake	7	1
Rice cake, mini, 1 cake	3	0
Rye cracker, 1 cracker	10	2
Saltine crackers, 1 cracker	2	0
Sunflower seeds, 1 tbsp	2	1
Tortilla chips, 12 chips or 13 strips	18	1
Tortilla chips, baked/low fat, 12 chips	22	2
Trail Mix (nuts/seeds/dried fruit), ¼ cup	18	5
Walnuts, ¼ cup	5	2
Wheat crackers, 1 cup	54	4
Whole wheat crackers, 1 cup	64	10
Zwieback crackers, 1 cracker	21	1
SWEETENERS/TOPPINGS		
Aspartame (EQUAL), 1 tsp	2	0
Aspartame (EQUAL), 1 packet	1	0
Baking chocolate, Semisweet Chocolate Mini Chips, 1 tbsp = 1 ounce	9	1
Caramel, 2 tbsp	30	0
Frosting, chocolate, 2 tbsp	26	0
Frosting, cream cheese-flavor, 2 tbsp	22	0
Frosting, French vanilla, 2 tbsp	25	0
Fructose, 1 tsp	4	0
Fructose, 1 tbsp	12	0
Glucose tablet, 1 "Dex"	4	0
Glucose tablet, 1 BD	5	0
Honey, 1 tsp	6	0
Honey, 1 tbsp	17	0
Jam/Jelly/Preserves, 1 tsp	5	0
Jam/Jelly/Preserves, 1 tbsp	16	0
Jam/Jelly/Preserves, low sugar, 1 tsp	2	0
Molasses, 1 tbsp	14	0
Sacharin (Sweet 'N Low), 1 packet	1	0
Splenda, 1 packet	0	0
Splenda, 1 tsp	1	0

	C	F
Sugar cube, ½" cube	6	0
Sugar Twin, 1 tsp	0	0
Sugar Twin, 1 packet	0	0
Sugar, Brown, 1 tbsp	13	0
Sugar, Brown, 1 tsp	4	0
Sugar, White, 1 tsp	3	0
Sugar, White, 1 tbsp	12	0
Syrup, average, 1 tbsp	14	0
Syrup, average, ¼ cup	55	0
Syrup, lite, 1 tbsp	6	0
Syrup, lite, ¼ cup	25	0

BAKED GOODS / PASTRY

	C	F
Angelfood cake, medium slice	25	0
animal crackers (includes arrowroot, tea biscuits), 1 oz	21	0
Biscotti, 1 small	10	0
Biscotti, 1 medium	20	0
Black Forest Cake, medium slice	34	1
Brownies, 2" by 3" piece	24	0
Butter cookie, 1 med	20	0
Cheesecake w/fruit topping, small slice	30	1
Cheesecake w/fruit topping, large slice	50	1
Cheesecake, plain, small slice	24	0
Cheesecake, plain, large slice	40	0
Chocolate chip cookie, 1 medium	15	1
Chocolate chip cookie, 1 small	7	0
Chocolate chip cookie, 1 large	38	0
Chocolate chip cookie, lower fat, 1 medium	21	1
Chocolate chip, soft-type, 1 medium	17	1
Chocolate sandwich, with creme filling (Oreo), 2 cookies	16	1
Chocolate sandwich, with double filling, 2 cookies	20	1
Cinnamon roll, medium (4 oz)	58	3
Cinnamon roll, large (6 oz)	87	5
Coconut macaroon cookie, 1 cookie	12	1
Coffee Cake w/crumb topping, medium slice	38	1

	C	F
Coffeecake, cheese, 1 oz	13	0
Cream puff, custard-filled, 1 medium	26	0
Croissant, small (1½ oz)	19	1
Croissant, medium (2 oz)	26	1
Croissant, large (2½ oz)	31	1
Cruller, glazed, 1 average	26	1
Cupcake with frosting, 1 average	30	1
Danish pastry, cheese, small slice	25	1
Danish pastry, fruit, small slice	28	1
Donut Holes, 1 average	8	0
Doughnut, glazed, 1 average	34	1
Doughnut w/icing, 1 average	29	1
Doughnut w/sugar topping, 1 average	27	1
Doughnut, plain, 1 average	25	1
Fig Newton, 2 cookies	22	2
Fruitcake, small slice	26	2
Funnel cake, 9"	85	0
Gingerbread, 3" square	37	2
Gingersnap, 1 small	6	0
Graham cracker, chocolate-coated, 1 square	19	1
Graham crackers, plain or honey, 1 square	6	0
Honey Bun, 1 average	47	2
Ice cream cones, cake or wafer-type, 1 cone	22	1
Ice cream cones, sugar, rolled-type, 1 cone	24	0
Lemon Cake, medium slice	40	1
Mallomar, 1 small	9	0
Meringue cookie, 1 small	5	0
Muffins: blueberry, corn, or oat bran, extra large (6 oz)	81	4
Muffins: blueberry, corn, or oat bran, large (5 oz)	67	4
Muffins: blueberry, corn, or oat bran, medium (4 oz)	54	3
Muffins: blueberry, corn, or oat bran, miniature	8	0
Muffins: blueberry, corn, or oat bran, small (2.5 oz)	32	2

	C	F
Oatmeal or oatmeal raisin cookie, 1 medium	15	1
Oatmeal raisin cookie, fat free, 1 medium	20	1
Peanut butter cookie, 1 small	7	0
Peanut butter cookie, 1 medium	14	1
Peanut Jumble, 1 cookie	13	1
Pie, apple, blueberry or cherry, large slice, ⅙ of 9" pie	69	1
Pie, apple, blueberry or cherry, small slice, ⅛ of 9" pie	46	1
Pie, chocolate cream, large slice, ⅙ of 9" pie	38	2
Pie, chocolate cream, small slice, ⅛ of 9" pie	30	2
Pie, cocount custard, large slice, ⅙ of 9" pie	31	2
Pie, cocount custard, small slice, ⅛ of 9" pie	25	2
Pie, Key Lime, ⅛ of 9" pie	43	2
Pie, Key Lime, ⅙ of 9" pie	54	2
Pie, lemon chiffon, large slice, ⅙ of 9" pie	50	1
Pie, lemon chiffon, small slice, ⅛ of 9" pie	40	1
Pie, lemon meringue, large slice, ⅙ of 9" pie	52	1
Pie, lemon meringue, small slice, ⅛ of 9" pie	42	1
Pie, pecan, large slice, ⅙ of 9" pie	59	4
Pie, pecan, small slice, ⅛ of 9" pie	47	4
Pie, pumpkin, large slice, ⅙ of 9" pie	30	3
Pie, pumpkin, small slice, ⅛ of 9" pie	24	3
Pineapple upside-down cake, medium slice	37	1
Pop Tart (Kellogg's), 1 average	37	1
Pop Tart (Kellogg's), low fat, 1 average	40	1
Pound cake, medium slice	42	0
Shortbread cookie, 1 small	5	0
Sponge cake, plain, medium slice	36	0
Strudel, toaster-size	26	1
Strudel, medium slice	45	1
Sugar cookie, 1 medium	17	0

	C	F
Sugar cookie, fat free, 1 med	17	0
Sweet Roll, small, 1 average	20	1
Vanilla sandwich cookie with creme filling, 1 oz	20	0
Vanilla wafers, 1 small	3	0
Vanilla wafers, lower fat, 1 small	3	0

MISC. DESSERTS

	C	F
Tapioca, home prepared, ½ cup	26	0
Cookie dough, refrigerated, ¼" slice	18	1
Bread pudding, ½ cup	40	1
Pudding, chocolate, ½ cup	26	0
Jell-O gelatin, ½ cup	18	0
Jell-O gelatin, sugar-free, ½ cup	0	0
Sherbet, ½ cup	28	0
Italian Ice, 1 cup	40	0
Ice Pops (frozen), single pop	10	0

CANDY

	C	F
Bon Bons, 1 piece	6	0
Candy corn, 24 pieces	37	0
Candy hearts (Necco), 1 small	2	0
Candy hearts (Necco), 1 large	4	0
Caramel, 1 piece	6	0
Chocloate-coated raisins, 30	21	1
Chocolate bar, average bar	23	1
Chocolate bar, king-size	42	2
Chocolate bar w/crisped rice, average bar	29	1
Chocolate bar w/crisped rice, king-size	51	2
Chocolate bar w/crisped rice, fun-size	7	0
Chocolate bar, w/almonds, average bar	20	2
Chocolate-coated pretzels, 3 mini	23	1
Chocolate-coated pretzels, 1 average	20	1
Chocolate miniatures, 1 piece	5	0
Chocolate-coated almonds, 6 pieces	11	1
Chocolate-coated peanuts, 12	15	1
Fruit Roll-Ups, 1 roll	20	0
Fudge, 1 oz	20	0

	C	F
Granola bar, soft, with peanut buttter & chocolate, 1 bar	20	1
Gum, average stick	2	0
Gum, 1 cube	6	0
Gum drops, 1 small	3	0
Gum drops, 1 large	7	0
Gum, small candy-coated, 1 piece	2	0
Gum, sugar-free, 1 piece	1	0
Gumball, 1 small	2	0
Gummi bears, 8	32	0
Gummi worms, 3	15	0
Hard candy, average, 1 piece	5	0
Hershey's Kiss, 1 piece	3	0
Jelly beans, 22 small	24	0
Jelly beans, 12 average	24	0
Lemon drops, 3	12	0
Licorice bites, 5	10	0
Licorice twist, 1 average	7	0
Life Savers, 1 average	2	0
Lollipop, small	6	0
Lollipop, 1 med	12	0
M & Ms, plain, 20 pieces	10	0
Malted milk balls, 10 pieces	16	0
Marshmallow, miniatures, ½ cup	24	0
Marshmallow, regular size, 5	23	0
Mints (after-dinner), chocolate & mint, 1 mint	3	0
Peanut Butter Cup, 1 miniature	4	0
Peanut Butter Cup, 1 average	12	1
Peppermint patties, chocolate covered, 1 small	11	0
Pixie, 1 piece	24	2
Rice Krispies Treat, 1 average	19	1
Salt Water Taffy, 5 pieces	34	0
Smarties, 1 roll	5	0
Snickers, regular bar	35	2
Snickers, 1 miniature	5	0
Toffee, 1 piece	5	0
Truffles, 1 regular piece	5	0

STARCH

HOT BREAKFAST	C	F
Pancake, plain, 4" diameter	11	1
Pancake, plain, 6" diameter	32	3
Waffle, frozen, 1 average	16	1
Waffle, homemade, 7"	26	1
French Toast, 1 slice	18	0
Grits, Corn/Hominy, cooked, 1 cup	31	1
Cream of Wheat, prepared, 1 cup	32	1
Oatmeal, instant, prepared with water, 1 cup	25	3

BREADS & BREAD PRODUCTS	C	F
Bagel Chips, 4 slices	17	1
Bagels, large, approx 4½" diameter	72	3
Bagels, medium, approx 3½-4" diameter	58	2
Bagels, mini, approx. 2½" diameter	16	1
Bagels, small, approx. 3" diameter	38	2
Biscuits, plain or buttermilk, 1 large	37	1
Biscuits, plain or buttermilk, 1 medium	25	1
Biscuits, plain or buttermilk, small	17	1
Bread crumbs, ¼ cup	20	1
Bread crumbs, 1 tbsp	6	0
Bread sticks, crunchy, medium, 7½" long	7	0
Bread sticks, crunchy, small, 4" long	3	0
Bread sticks, fresh baked, 1 medium	20	0
Bread, banana, 1 medium slice	33	1
Bread, cornbread, dry mix, prepared, 1 medium piece	29	1
Bread, cracked-wheat, 1 slice	12	1
Bread, egg (challah), 1 slice	19	1
Bread, french or vienna (includes sourdough) large, approx. 6" x 2½" x 1¾" slice	50	3
Bread, french or vienna (includes sourdough) medium, approx. 4" x 2½" x 1¾" slice	33	2
Bread, french or vienna (includes sourdough) small, approx. 2" x 2½" x 1¾" slice	17	1
Bread, Irish soda, 1 slice	16	1

	C	F
Bread, Italian large slice (1.1 ounce), approx. 4½" x 3¼" x ¾" slice	15	1
Bread, Italian small slice, approx. 3¼" x 2½" x ½" slice	5	0
Bread, light/reduced calorie, average, 1 oz	7	1
Bread, mixed-grain, 1 slice	15	2
Bread, oat bran, 1 slice	12	1
Bread, oatmeal, 1 slice	13	1
Bread, pumpernickel, 1 slice	13	2
Bread, raisin, 1 slice	15	1
Bread, rye, 1 slice	14	2
Bread, wheat, 1 slice	13	1
Bread, white, 1 slice	15	1
Bread, white, commercially prepared (includes soft bread crumbs), 1 cup, crumbs	23	1
Bread, whole wheat, 1 slice	13	2
Cracker meal, 1 cup	93	3
Croutons, plain or seasoned average, ¼ cup	6	0
English muffin, average, 2 oz	27	1
Pita, large whole wheat, 6½" diameter	35	5
Pita, large, white, 6½" diameter	33	1
Pita, small, white, 4" diameter	16	1
Pita, small, whole wheat, 4" diameter	15	2
Rolls, dinner-type, 2½" diameter, 1 roll	18	1
Rolls, dinner-type, 3½" diameter, 1 roll	23	1
Rolls, hamburger, 1 roll	23	0
Rolls, hard (kaiser), 3½" diameter, 1 roll	30	1
Rolls, hoagie/submarine/grinder/hero, 6" long	45	0
Rolls, hoagie/submarine/grinder/hero, 10" long	75	0
Rolls, hot dog, 1 roll	19	0
Rolls, hot dog, footlong, 1 roll	43	0
Matzo, Passover, 1 square sheet	27	1
Matzo, regular, 1 square sheet	22	1
Noodles, crunchy chow mein-style, 1 cup	26	2

	C	F
Stuffing, prepared, ½ cup	11	0
Taco shells, large (6½" diameter), 1 shell	13	2
Taco shells, medium (5" diameter), 1 shell	8	1
Taco shells, mini (3" diameter), 1 shell	3	0
Tortilla, corn, 6"	9	0
Tortilla, flour, large (burrito-size), 12"	32	0
Tortilla, flour, medium (fajita-size), 10"	25	0
Tortilla, flour, small (taco-size), 6"	15	0

CEREALS

	C	F
Bran flakes, ¾ cup	24	5
Cornflakes, 1 cup	24	1
Crisp rice, 1 cup	21	0
Farina, cooked, 1 cup	24	1
Frosted corn flakes, 1 cup	35	1
Granola, ⅔ cup	44	3
Grape Nuts, ½ cup	47	5
Oat bran flakes, 1 cup	37	6
Puffed rice, 1 cup	14	0
Puffed wheat, 1 cup	12	1
Raisin Bran, 1 cup	47	7
Shredded wheat, 2 biscuits	36	6
Shredded wheat (bite-size), 1 cup	41	6
Toasted Oats (Cheerios), 1 cup	22	4
Wheat flakes, 1 cup	24	3
Wheat germ, toasted, 1 cup	56	17

GRAINS

	C	F
Bulgur, cooked, 1 cup	34	8
Corn: see vegetables section		
Cornmeal, whole grain, 1 cup	94	9
Cornstarch, 1 cup	117	1
Couscous, cooked, 1 cup	36	2
Lentils, cooked, 1 cup	40	16
Matzo meal, 1 cup	110	4
Millet, cooked, 1 cup	41	2
Millet, puffed, 1 cup	17	1
Oat bran, cooked, 1 cup	25	6

	C	F
Potatoes: see vegetables section		
Quinoa, cooked, ½ cup	17	2
Rice bran, crude, 1 cup	59	25
Rice noodles, cooked, 1 cup	44	2
Rice pilaf, 1 cup	43	2
Rice, brown, cooked, 1 cup	45	4
Rice, fried (Chinese-style), 1 cup	42	1
Rice, white, instant, cooked, 1 cup	53	1
Rice, white, long-grain, cooked, 1 cup	45	1
Risotto, 1 cup	65	2
Semolina, 1 cup	122	7
Wheat germ, ¼ cup	15	4
Wheat, sprouted, 1 cup	46	1
Wild rice, cooked, 1 cup	35	3

FLOUR

	C	F
Barley, 1 cup	110	15
Arrowroot, 1 cup	113	4
Buckwheat, 1 cup	85	12
Carob, 1 cup	92	41
Chickpea (besan), 1 cup	53	10
Corn, enriched or whole grain, 1 cup	89	13
Corn, unenriched, 1 cup	104	2
Potato, 1 cup	133	9
Rice, brown, 1 cup	121	7
Rice, white, 1 cup	127	4
Rye, dark, 1 cup	88	29
Rye, light or medium, 1 cup	80	15
Soy, defatted, 1 cup	36	17
Soy, full or low fat, 1 cup	30	8
Wheat, white, 1 cup	95	3
Wheat, whole grain, 1 cup	87	15

BEANS

	C	F
Beans, adzuki cooked, 1 cup	57	17
Beans, baked, 1 cup	50	10
Beans, black turtle soup, cooked, 1 cup	40	17
Beans, black, cooked, 1 cup	41	15
Beans, chili, cooked, 1 cup	43	11

	C	F
Beans, cranberry (roman), cooked, 1 cup	42	17
Beans, fava (broad beans), cooked, 1 cup	33	9
Beans, french, cooked, 1 cup	43	17
Beans, great northern, cooked, 1 cup	43	13
Beans, kidney, cooked, 1 cup	40	15
Beans, lima, ½ cup	17	4
Beans, Mung, cooked, 1 cup	36	14
Beans, navy, cooked, average, 1 cup	49	17
Beans, pinto, cooked, 1 cup	42	14
Beans, refried, 1 cup	39	13
Beans, snap, green or yellow, cooked, raw, or frozen, average, 1 cup	8	4
Chickpeas (garbanzo beans), cooked, 1 cup	48	12
Chili con carne with beans, canned entree, 1 cup	29	11
Succotash (corn and limas), cooked, 1 cup	37	7

PASTA

	C	F
Macaroni, cooked, 1 cup	43	3
Macaroni, cooked, vegetable or whole wheat, 1 cup	37	5
Noodles, egg, cooked, 1 cup	40	2
Pasta (general): linguini, tortellini, ravioli, fettucini, 1 cup	37	2
Pasta shells, cooked, 1 cup	31	2
Spaghetti, plain or spinach, cooked, 1 cup	37	2
Spaghetti, whole wheat, cooked, 1 cup	37	6
Tortellini, pasta with cheese filling, ¾ cup	38	2

VEGETABLES

	C	F
Alfalfa seeds, sprouted, raw, 1 cup	1	1
Artichokes (Jerusalem), raw, ½ cup	13	1
Artichokes, (globe or French), cooked, ½ cup	9	5

	C	F
Artichokes, (globe or French), raw, ½ cup	11	5
Arugula, raw, 1 leaf	0	0
Asparagus, boiled, drained, ½ cup	4	2
Asparagus, raw, 1 cup	5	3
Avocado, raw, ½, medium	6	4
Avocados, raw, California, ½ cup	10	8
Balsam pear (bitter gourd), leafy tips, 1 cup	4	1
Balsam pear (bitter gourd), pods cooked, 1 cup	5	2
Balsam pear (bitter gourd), pods, raw, 1 cup	3	3
Bamboo shoots, cooked, 1 cup	2	1
Bamboo shoots, raw, 1 cup	8	3
Beans, snap, cooked, 1 cup	10	4
Beans, snap, raw, 1 cup	8	4
Beets, cooked, 1 cup	16	4
Beets, raw, 1 cup	13	4
Broccoli raab, cooked, 1 bunch	14	12
Broccoli raab, raw, 1 cup	4	0
Broccoli, cooked, ½ cup	4	2
Broccoli, raw, ½ cup	2	1
Brussels sprouts boiled, ½ cup	7	3
Brussels sprouts, raw, ½ cup	4	2
Cabbage, cooked, ½ cup	3	2
Cabbage, raw, ½ cup	2	1
Carrot juice, 6 oz	14	2
Carrots, baby, raw, 10 pieces	8	2
Carrots, cooked, ½ cup	8	3
Carrots, raw, ½ cup	6	2
Cauliflower, cooked or raw, ½ cup	3	2
Celery, cooked or raw, ½ cup	3	1
Celtuce, raw, 10 leaves	4	2
Chard, Swiss, raw or cooked, ½ cup	3	1
Chicory greens, raw, ½ cup	4	4
Chicory, witloof, raw, ½ cup	2	1
Chrysanthemum, garland, boiled, 1 cup	4	2
Chrysanthemum, garland, raw, 1 cup	1	1
Coleslaw, ½ cup	7	0
Collards, boiled, 1 cup	8	3
Collards, raw, 1 cup	2	1
Corn on cob, white or yellow, 1 large ear	22	2
Corn, whole kernel, canned, ½ cup	15	2
Cress, garden, raw, ½ cup	1	0
Cress, garden, boiled, ½ cup	3	1
Cucumber, raw, ½ cup	2	1
Dandelion greens, boiled, 1 cup	7	3
Dandelion greens, raw, 1 cup	5	2
Eggplant, boiled, 1 cup	9	2
Eggplant, pickled, 1 cup	13	3
Eggplant, raw, 1 cup	5	3
Endive, raw, 1 head	17	16
Fungi, Cloud ears, dried, ½ cup	10	10
Hummus, ½ cup	22	12
Jute, potherb, boiled, 1 cup	6	2
Kale, boiled or raw, 1 cup	7	2
Kohlrabi, boiled, 1 cup	11	2
Kohlrabi, raw, 1 cup	8	5
Leeks, (bulb and lower leaf portion), boiled, 1 leek	9	1
Leeks, (bulb and lower leaf portion), raw, 1 cup	13	2
Lettuce, romaine, green leaf, red leaf, or iceberg, 1 cup	1	1
Lotus root, boiled, 1 cup	20	4
Lotus root, raw, 10 slices	14	4
Mushroom, oyster, raw, 1 large	10	4
Mushrooms, white, portabella, raw, or stir fried, average, 1 cup	3	1
Mustard greens, boiled or raw, average, 1 cup	3	2
Mustard spinach, (tendergreen), raw or boiled, 1 cup	6	0
Okra, boiled or raw, ½ cup	7	3
Olives (black), 1 medium	0.5	0
Olives (green), 1 medium	0	0
Onions, dehydrated flakes, 1 tbsp	4	0
Onions, green (includes tops and bulb), raw, 1 cup	7	3
Onions, green, tops only, 1 tbsp	0	0
Onions, sweet, raw, 1 cup	16	2
Onions, yellow, sauteed, 1 cup	7	1

	C	F
Peas in pod, raw, ½ cup	4	2
Peas, green, boiled, ½ cup	13	5
Peas, green, raw, 1 cup	21	7
Pepper, ancho, dried, 1 pepper	9	4
Peppers, hot chili, green, raw, 1 pepper	4	1
Peppers, hot chili, red, raw, 1 pepper	4	1
Peppers, jalapeno, raw, ½ cup	4	2
Peppers, sweet, green, raw, 1 cup	7	3
Peppers, sweet, red, raw, 1 cup	9	3
Peppers, sweet, yellow, raw, 1 pepper	12	2
Potato pancakes, 1 small	6	1
Potato salad, 1 cup	35	3
Potato skin only, 1 medium	27	5
Potato, baked, medium	63	7
Potato, russet, baked, large	80	5
Potato, russet, baked, medium	64	7
Potato, russet, baked, small	31	2
Potatoes, au gratin, 1 cup	28	4
Potatoes, boiled, with skin, 1 cup	32	4
Potatoes, French Fried, small serving	28	
Potatoes, French Fried, medium serving	45	
Potatoes, French Fried, large serving	65	
Potatoes, French Fried, 1 cup	60	
Potatoes, hashed brown, 1 cup	55	5
Potatoes, mashed, 1 cup	35	3
Potatoes, scalloped, 1 cup	31	3
Pumpkin, mashed, 1 cup	12	3
Radicchio, raw, 1 cup	2	0
Radishes, pickled, 1 cup	8	3
Radishes, raw, average, 1 cup, slices	3	2
Rutabagas, boiled, 1 cup, mashed	21	0
Rutabagas, raw, 1 cup	11	4

	C	F
Seaweed, kelp, raw, 2 tbsp	1	0
Seaweed, spirulina, dried, 1 cup	4	1
Seeds, assorted, 1 tsp	1	0
Spices, assorted, 1 tsp	1	0
Spinach souffle, 1 cup	8	1
Spinach, boiled, 1 cup	7	4
Spinach, raw, 1 cup	1	1
Squash, summer, all varieties, cooked, 1 cup	7	3
Squash, summer, all varieties, raw, 1 cup	4	1
Squash, winter, all varieties, cooked, 1 cup	20	6
Squash, winter, all varieties, raw, 1 cup	15	2
Succotash, (corn and limas), raw, ½ cup	23	4
Sweet potato, baked, medium	24	4
Sweet potato, cooked, candied, home-prepared, 1 piece	29	3
Sweet potato, mashed, 1 cup	58	8
Taro leaves, raw, 1 cup	2	1
Taro, leaves, steamed, 1 cup	6	3
Tomato, medium	6	2
Tomato, medium slice	1	0
Tomato (cherry), 1	1	0
Tomato juice, 6 oz	5	0
Tomatoes, grape, 3	2	0
Tomatoes, sun-dried, 1 cup	30	7
Turnip greens, boiled, 1 cup	6	5
Turnip greens, raw, 1 cup	4	2
Vegetable juice, 8 oz	10	1
Waterchestnuts, raw, ½ cup, slices	15	2
Watercress, raw, 1 cup, chopped	0	0
Yam, boiled, 1 cup	38	5

Eating "Out"

Ethnic Foods

African

SOUPS/STEWS	C	F
Bean Soup (Gbegiri), 1 cup	13	0
Beef & Vegetable Soup, 1 cup	6	1
Fish Soup (Alapa), 1½ cups	4	0
Okra Soup, 1½ cups	6	1
Sunday Stew, 1½ cups	8	1

SIDE DISHES	C	F
Black-Eyed Bean Fritters (Kosai-akara), 2 1-inch fritters	13	1
Boiled Sweet Potatoes w/peanuts (Dankali da geda), 1 cup	51	3
Coconut and Sweet Corn, ¾ cup	20	4
Couscous, 1 cup	45	3
Fufu Cornmeal (Ine-oka), 1 cup	88	1
Fufu Rice (Rice Tuwo), 1 cup	57	0
Fufu Yam Flour, 1 cup	88	2
Plantains, Deep Fried (Ipekere), ½ plantain	24	1

MAIN DISHES	C	F
Curried meat triangles, 2	7	0
Chopone-Choptwo triangles, 2	8	0
Pepper Chicken, 1 breast	3	0
Pork Pineapple, 8 oz	16	1
Stuffed vegetables, 8 oz	10	1

DESSERTS	C	F
Banana Fritters, 1 cup	42	1
Mango slice, 1 cup	57	1
Niger Pineapple, 1 cup	43	0
Pawpaw Fool, 1 cup	32	1

Cajun & Creole

APPETIZERS & SIDES	C	F
Bouillabaisse, 1 cup	10	0
Cocktail Sauce, 2 Tbsp	6	0
Couche-couche, ½ cup	17	0
Crawfish Bisque, 1 serving	10	0

	C	F
Hogshead Cheese, ½ cup	0	0
Red Beans & Rice, 1 cup	52	8
Remoulade Sauce, 2 Tbsp, 1 oz	2	0

MAIN DISHES	C	F
Alligator, 4 oz cooked	0	0
Baked Herb Chicken, 1 serving	2	0
Cajun Fried Turkey, 1 serving	0	0
Crawfish, cooked, 4 oz	0	0
Creole Jambalaya, 1 serving	15	
Frog's Legs, steamed (2)	0	0
Guinea Fowl, flesh, 4 oz, ckd	0	0
Jambalaya, Shrimp & Crabmeat	12	0
Roasted Quail, w. Bacon on Toast	15	1
Shrimp Creole, 1 serving	10	0
Stuffed Smothered Steak, w. 1 cup Rice	30	1
Turtle, cooked, 3 oz	0	0

Caribbean

APPETIZERS	C	F
Banana fritters, 1 cup	29	1
Plantain chips, 1 cup	47	1
Shrimp fritters, 1 cup	20	0

SOUPS & SIDES	C	F
Black Beans and Rice, 1½ cups	50	1
Callaloo Soup, 1 cup	15	1
Calabaza (Colombo de Giraumon), 1 cup	23	2
Shrimp Bisque, 1 cup	11	0

MAIN DISHES	C	F
Chicken Stew (Sanocho), 1½ cups	26	1
Lamb w/Beans & Rice, 1½ cups	51	1
Stuffed Plantains (Piononos), 2 4-oz patties	42	1
White Fish in Broth (Blaff), 8 oz	6	0

	C	F
Crayfish (Ouassous au nage), 1½ cups	10	0

DESSERTS

	C	F
Key Lime Pie, 4" slice	59	0
Mango Fritters, 2	22	1

BEVERAGES

	C	F
Daiquiri/Banana, 1 cup	23	0
Daquiri/Strawberry, 1 cup	35	1
Ginger Beer, 1 cup	12	0
Planter's Punch, ¾ cup	24	0

Chinese

APPETIZERS

	C	F
Barbecued Sparerib, 1	13	0
Crab Puff/Rangoon, 1	7	0
Curried meat triangles, 1	12	0
Dumplings steamed (shrimp/pork), 1	10	0
Dumplings steamed (vegetable), 1	3	0
Egg Roll (medium), 1	21	1
Egg Roll (mini), 1	4	0
Rice paper roll, 1	10	0
Spring Roll, 1	11	0
Wonton (fried), 1	5	0

SOUPS

	C	F
Clear Soup w/Noodles, 1 bowl	12	0
Clear Soup, 1 bowl	4	0
Egg Drop Soup w/out Noodles, 1cup	3	0
Egg Drop Soup: w. Noodles, 1 cup	15	0
Hot & Sour Soup, 1 cup	5	0
Shark Fin Soup, 1 cup	4	0
Sizzling Rice Soup, 1 cup	31	0
Velvet Corn Soup, 1 cup	18	1
Winter Melon Soup, 1 cup	8	0
Wonton Soup, 1 cup	19	0

MAIN DISHES

	C	F
Beef in Black Bean Sauce, 17 oz	17	1
Beef with Broccoli, 1 cup	4	0
Beef: shredded, hot & spicy, 1 cup	15	1
Black Sea Bass steamed, 8 oz	1	0

	C	F
Buddha's Delight vegetables, 1 cup	9	1
Chicken (sliced) & Broccoli, 1 cup	13	2
Chicken w/cashews, 1 cup	12	0
Chop Suey: Pork, 2 cups	10	1
Chop Suey: Chicken, 2 cups	6	1
Clams with Black Bean Sauce, 9 clams	6	0
Crispy Fried Chicken, 8 oz	12	1
Drunken Chicken, 8 oz	12	0
Duck braised, 1¾ cups	23	1
Green Beans (spicy), ¾ cup	7	1
Kung Pao Chicken, 1 cup	16	1
Kung Pao Shrimp, 1 cup	20	1
Lemon Chicken, 8 oz	2	0
Mu Shu Pork, 2 wrapped crepes	35	1
Omelet, Chicken/Shrimp, 6 oz	10	9
Orange beef, 1 cup	20	0
Shrimp w/Lobster Sauce, 7 oz	8	0
Steamed Whole Fish, Red Snapper, 8 oz	1	0
Sweet & Sour: Cabbage, ½ cup	18	1
Sweet & Sour: Chicken, 1¼ cups	43	1
Sweet & Sour: Pork, 2 cups	74	1
Vegetable Combination (stir fried), ⅔ cup	15	1

RICE/NOODLES DISHES

	C	F
Chow Mein, Beef/Chicken, 1¼ cups	37	2
Egg Foo Yong w/Sauce, 1 cup	11	2
Fried Rice, 1 cup	42	0
Lo Mein (pork), 1½ cups	83	0
Lo Mein (vegetable), 1½ cups	85	1
Noodles cooked, 1 cup	42	2
Rice: plain brown/steamed, 1 cup	76	1
Rice: plain white/steamed, 1 cup	78	0

SAUCES

	C	F
Duck Sauce, 2 tbsp	23	0
Mustard Sauce, 2 tbsp	4	0
Peanut Sauce/Dip, 2 tbsp	5	0
Spicy Dipping Sauce, 2 tbsp	3	0

DESSERTS	C	F
Almond Cookie, 1	6	0
Fortune Cookie, 1	6	0
Sorbet, ½ cup	14	0

BEVERAGES	C	F
Bubble Tea, average, 12 fl oz	55	0

Cuban

APPETIZERS/SIDES	C	F
Blk.-eyed Pea Fritters (Bollitos de Carita), each	6	
Cuban Bread (Pan Cubano), 1 slice	15	

MAIN DISHES	C	F
Black Beans w. Rice (Morns con Cfistianos), 1½ cups	76	12
Corn Tamale Casserole, 1 cup	55	4
Chicken w. Yellow Rice (Arroz con Pollo), 2 cups	87	4
Roast Pork Sandwich (Pan con Lechon), 1	62	2
Seasoned Beef w. Olives & Raisins (Picadillo), 1 cup	10	2
Shredded Beef (Ropa Vieja), 1 cup	10	0
Taro Root Mash (Pure de Malanga), 1 cup	69	4
Yuca with Citrus Garlic Dressing (Yuca con Mojo), 1 cup	25	1

DESSERTS	C	F
Donut in Syrup (Bunuelos), small	10	0
Grilled Plantains, 2	40	8
Gypsy's Arm Cake (Brazo Gitano), 1 slice	42	1

French

APPETIZERS/SOUPS	C	F
Escargots (Snails), garlic butter (6)	4	0
French Onion Soup, 1½ cups	15	0
Potage Creme Crecy (Carrot Soup), 1 cup	14	2
Salade Nicoise (Tuna/Oliv./Veg.)	14	1
Vichyssoise (Pot./leek Soup), 1 cup	15	1

MAIN DISHES	C	F
Blanquette d'Agneau (Lamb Stew), 1 cup	17	0
Bouillabaisse (Fish Stew), 1 cup	13	0
Burgundy Beef Stew (Boeuf Bourguignon), 1 cup	26	2
Coq au Vin (Chicken in Wine), 2 cups	11	1
Coquilles St. Jacgues, fried, 6 large	2	0
Duck a l'Orange, 13 oz	29	1
Frogs Legs, fried, 4 med. pairs	10	1
Lamb Noisettes, fried, 2 chops	1	0
Onion Tart, 6 oz	17	0
Quiceh Lorraine, 6 oz	16	0
Rack of Lamb (Carre d'Agneau Vert Pre), ½ rack	0	0
Salmon fillets, 8 oz	3	0
Veal Cordon Bleu (Veal/Ham/Ch)	18	0
Veal Scallops (sauteed), 8 oz	3	1
White Bean Casserole (Cassoulet), 2 cups	32	2

SIDES & SAUCES	C	F
Bearnaise Sauce, ¼ cup	1	0
Bechamel Sauce, ⅓ cup	11	0
Broiled Tomatoes (Tomatoes a la Provencale), 5 oz	5	0
French Stick Bread, 3 slices	35	3
Hollandaise Sauce, ¼ cup	0	0
Mornay Sauce, ¼ cup	5	0
Mushroom Stuffing w/Shallots, ⅓ cup	4	1
Mushrooms marinated, 5 oz	6	2
Potatoes in Cream, 5 oz	27	1
Ratatoille Nicoise, 1¾ cups	22	2

DESSERTS	C	F
Chocolate Genoise, ½ cup	46	0
Chocolate Mousse, ¼ cup	11	0
Creme Brulee, 1 serving	21	0
Creme Caramel (Caramel Custard), ½ cup	29	0
Crepe Suzette w/Sauce, 6" crepe	13	0
Mousse au Chocolat, ½ cup	33	0

	C	F
Napoleon, medium	75	1
Rum Cake, 1 slice	39	0
Tarte Tatin, 1 cup	49	1

German

SOUPS & SIDES

	C	F
Cabbage Soup, 1 cup	3	0
Dumpling, 3 small	28	0
Herring, Pickled: ½ cup	3	0
Potato Salad, ¾ cup	20	1
Potato Soup, 1 cup	12	0
Sauerkraut, ¾ cup	10	2
Spatzle, ½ cup	43	0

MAIN DISHES

	C	F
Beef Goulash with Vegetables, 2 cups	46	2
Bratwurst, grilled, 1 medium, 6 oz	2	0
Chicken: Fried, Viennese-style	28	1
Hot Sausage Curry	6	0
Knockwurst, 1 medium	2	0
Liver w. Apple/Onion, 6 oz	10	1
Liverwurst, 1 oz	1	0
Pork Chops with Saurkraut, 1 chop	21	2
Rabbit Stew, 6 oz	8	0
Sauerbraten Pork (Pot Roast), 8 oz	15	0
Veal Paprikash, 8 oz	7	0
Weiner Schnitzel, 1 medium	5	0

DESSERTS

	C	F
Apple Strudel, 2" slice	37	1
Black Forest Cake, 1 slice	30	0
Kugelhupf Cake, 1 slice	40	0
Sachertorte glazed, 2" slice	53	0
Torte: Linzer, 3" wedge	41	1

Greek

APPETIZERS & SALADS

	C	F
Baba Ghanouj, 1 tbsp	2	0
Calamari, deep fried, 1 cup	17	0
Chicken-Lemon Soup, 1 cup	12	0
Hummus, 1 tbsp	7	1

	C	F
Pita Bread, 8" round	26	0
Soup: Argolemono (Egg Lemon Soup w/ Chicken & Rice), 1 cup	5	0
Spanakopita, 3" square	11	0
Tabbouleh, 1 cup	22	0
Taramasalata, 1 tbsp	2	0
Tzatziki (Cucumber/Yog. Dip), 1 tbsp	3	0
Vine Leaves, stuffed (Dolmas), 8 small rolls	17	1

MAIN DISHES

	C	F
Chicken Kebob, 1	8	0
Gyros meat, 4 oz	6	0
Gyros on Pita w/Sauce	42	2
Hummus & Pita, 4 oz	30	6
Greek Chicken Salad, ½ cup	9	1
Moussaka, 8 oz	22	2
Pastitsio, 12 oz	19	1
Souvlakia (Lamb), 2 oz	1	0
Stuffed Tomatoes, 2	17	3
Tahini, 1 tbsp	2	1

DESSERTS

	C	F
Galactobureko, (Filo, Custard, Pastry in Syrup), 1	48	0
Baklava Pastry, large	45	0
Baklava Pastry, small	32	0
Halva, 2 oz piece	23	1
Kataifi (Filo, Nut, Pastry in Syrup), 1	56	1
Turkish Delight, 2" square	35	2
Tyropita (Filo/Egg/Cheese Pastry), 1	31	0

Hawaiian

APPETIZERS / SIDE DISHES

	C	F
Gyoza, Potsticker Dumplings, 1 only	6	0
Haupia (Coconut Pudding), 1 piece	17	0
Hawaiian Sweet Bread, ½" slice	29	2
Kirn Chee (pickled cabbage), ½ cup	5	1
Manapua Dumplings, (Char Siu Pork Bun)	25	0
Poi (mashed cooked taro), 1 cup	65	

	C	F
Poke, Fish Salad, average all types, 3 oz	0	0
Spam Musubi	34	0

MAIN DISHES

	C	F
Ahi Tuna (grilled), 6 oz fillet	0	0
Kalua Chicken, 4 oz	0	0
Kalua Pork, 4oz	0	0
LauLau Chicken, 7 oz	3	0
Laulau Pork, 7oz	5	0
Loco Moco (rice/burger/egg/gravy)	63	2
Lomi Salmon, ¼ cup	2	0
Taro Pancake Mix, ⅓ cup	26	2

DESSERTS

	C	F
Kulolo (Taro Pudding), 1 slice	19	1
Malasadas (Donut), 1	26	0
Shave Ice (Mateumoto), all flavors: w. Beans, 1 large	72	4
Shave Ice (Mateumoto), all flavors: w. Ice cream, 1 large	64	0

Indian & Pakistani

APPETIZERS & SIDES

	C	F
Chapati/Roti, 7" diam. piece	11	0
Chutney (mango), ½ cup	25	1
Cucumber Raita, ½ cup	4	0
Mulligatawney Soup, 1 cup	8	0
Naan Bread, 8" x 2"	11	0
Poori, 3"	7	0

MAIN DISHES

	C	F
Alu Gosht Kari (Meat/Pot. Curry)	23	0
Chicken Biriyani, 1 cup	63	0
Chicken Korma, 2 oz	6	0
Chicken Pilaf (Murgh Biriyani), 1 cup	50	4
Chicken Tikka, 3 short skewers	3	0
Chicken Vindaloo, 1 cup	5	0
Curried Garbanzo Beans, ½ cup	33	3
Curry mixed vegetable, 1½ cups	20	2
Dal (Lentil Puree): 1 cup	37	14
Dhakla (Lentil Dish), 1" square	13	3

	C	F
Fish w/Cilantro & Chili, 9 oz	7	0
Gosht Kari (Meat Curry/Tom./Pot.), 1 cup	17	2
Lamb Pilaf, 1½ cups	40	1
Lentils spiced brown, ¾ cup	18	1
Okra spicy, 1 cup	11	1
Pesrattu (Lentil Crepe), 9", 2.6 oz	15	3
Pork Vindaloo Curry	3	0
Rajmah (Kidney Bean Curry), 1 cup	35	13
Saffron Rice, 1 cup	71	0
Shahi Korma (Braised Lamb), 1¼ cups	8	1
Shrimp and Mustard Seeds, 4 oz	2	0
Tandoori Chicken: Breast	5	0
Tandoori Chicken: Leg/Thigh portion	6	0

DESSERTS

	C	F
Cardamom and Nut Ice Cream, ½ cup	29	0
Pistachio Halva, 2" square	7	0
Saffron Rice Pudding, 1 cup	66	0

Italian

APPETIZERS

	C	F
Breadstick (Cheese), 1	20	0
Breadstick, 1	25	0
Broccoli Rabe, ½ cup	5	1
Bruschetta, 2 slices	23	2
Caponata, ¾ cup	8	1
Eggplant & Zucchini (fried), ½ cup	10	0
Eggplant Salad (marinated), ⅓ cup	2	0
Focaccia with Rosemary and Garlic, ½ cup	29	0
Garlic Bread, 6" long	24	0
Mushrooms (marinated), 1/3 cup	2	1
Olives (marinated), ½ cup	3	1
Peppers (roasted), ½ cup	2	0
Pizaa Margherita, small slice	30	0
Provolone (fried), ½ cup	8	0

SOUPS & SALADS

	C	F
Caesar Salad, 1½ cups	11	1

	C	F
Calamari Salad, ¾ cup	17	1
Minestrone (Genoa style), 1 cup	16	1
Minestrone (Neapolitan), 1 cup	9	1
Pastina and Egg soup, 1 cup	6	0
Spinach Salad, 1½ cups	6	1
Tuscan Bean soup, 1 cup	10	1

MAIN DISHES

Baked Ziti, 1¾ cups	82	2
Calzone, average	101	2
Cannelloni, 1 lg tube	18	0
Chicken Cacciatora, 2 pieces chicken	7	1
Chicken Marsala, 2 pieces chicken	9	0
Chicken Parmigiana, 2 breasts	16	0
Eggplant Parmesan, 2 cups	33	3
Fettucine Alfredo, 1 cup	47	0
Fettucine Prosciutto, 1 cup	51	1
Fish Stew, 2½ cups	30	1
Gnocchi (potato), 1 cup	44	1
Gnocchi Alla Romana, 1 cup	12	1
Lasagne, 1 cup	45	1
Linguine w/Clam Sauce, 1 cup	56	0
Meatballs in Mushroom Sauce, 2 medium	13	3
Pasta Primavera, 1½ cups	51	1
Pizza: Deep Dish, ⅙ medium (11")	57	2
Pizza: Deep Dish, Personal (6"), whole	58	2
Pizza: Per Slice ⅛ medium (11"), Thick Crust	29	1
Pizza: Per Slice ⅛ medium, (11"), Thin Crust	21	1
Polenta, 10 oz	34	1
Ravioli, 1½ cups	75	2
Rigatoni (baked), 1¾ cups	28	1
Risoto Milanese, 1¼ cups	48	0
Shrimp Scampi, 4 shrimp	2	0
Spaghetti Carbonara, 1¼ cups	55	0
Spaghetti w. Meat Sauce, 2 cups	74	0
Spaghetti w. Meatballs, 1½ cups	57	1

DESSERTS

	C	F
Lemon Ice, 1 cup	45	0
Biscotti, 2	23	0
Biscuit Tortoni, 3 oz	12	1
Risotto Pudding, 1¼ cups	92	1
Spumoni, ½ cup	25	0
Tiramisu, ⅔ cup	16	0
Zabaglione, ¼ cup	10	0

Japanese

SOUP, SALAD, APPETIZERS

Edamame (young green soybeans): (no pods), ½ cup	12	4
Edamame (young green soybeans): (in pods), ½ cup	5	2
Miso Soup w. Tofu pieces, 1 cup	11	1
Mushroom Soup (clear), 1 cup	4	1
Seaweed Salad, 1 cup	0	0

SUSHI

Futomaki (hand roll), 4 oz	18	0
Futomaki (thick roll), 6 pieces	72	1
Inari (rice filled soybean pocket), 4 pieces	73	3
Sashimi (Sliced Raw Seafood or Beef), 1 piece	0	0
Sushi (Maki) Rolls large 2¼" diam. - per piece	9	0
Sushi (Maki) Rolls medium 1¾" diam. - per piece	7	0
Sushi (Maki) Rolls small 1 1/8" diam. - per piece	4	0
Sushi Rice: cooked, 1 Cup	82	2
Sushi-Nigiri (fish on rice): 1 average piece	12	0

MAIN DISHES

Prawns in the shell, 2 large shrimp	1	0
Soba Noodles, 1 cup	43	2
Sukiyaki(Beef/Tofu/Veg.), 2 cups	19	1
Tempura (Batter-fried Shrimp or Vegetable), 1 piece	7	0
Teppanyaki (Steak, Seafood & Vegetables)	15	1
Teriyaki: Beef, 4 oz serving	4	0
Teriyaki: Chicken, 4 oz serving	7	0
Teriyaki: Salmon, 6 oz serving	3	0

	C	F
Teriyaki: Shrimp, 6 oz serving	4	0
Yakatori, 1 skewer	1	0

MISCELLANEOUS

	C	F
Bean Curd Tofu, 6 oz	4	1
Ginger Vinegar Dressing, 2 Tbsp	6	0
Sake Wine (16% alc.), 3 oz	7	0
Soy Sauce, 2 tbsp	3	0
Tempura Sauce, ½ cup	8	0
Teriyaki Sauce, 2 tbsp	11	0
Wasabi, ½ tsp	2	0

Kosher & Deli Foods

SOUPS

	C	F
Borscht: (no cream), 1 cup	14	3
Borscht: Diet/Reduced Cal, 1 cup	7	2
Chicken Broth: 1 cup	0	0
Chicken Broth: with vegetables, 1 cup	5	0
Chicken Broth: with noodles, 1 cup	16	0
Matzo Ball Soup: ¾ cup w. 2 small or 1 large ball	27	1
Matzo Ball Soup: Bowl (approx. 1½ Cups) with Chicken& Noodles	34	1
Schmaltz (Rendered chicken fat), 1 tbsp	0	0

BREADS

	C	F
Bagel/Bialy, 1 small, 2 oz	32	1
Bagel/Bialy, 1 medium, 4 oz	64	2
Bagel/Bialy, 1 large, 5 oz	80	3
Challah bread, 1 slice	14	1
Mandelbrot (Almond Bread), 1 slice, ¼" thick	5	0

MAIN DISHES

	C	F
Cabbage Roll (meat/rice), 5 oz	21	1
Chopped Liver with Egg Salad, ¼ cup	3	0
Chopped Liver: ¼ cup	5	0
Herring: Smoked in Sour Cream, ¼ cup	0	0
Herring: Smoked, ¼ cup	0	0
Lox (Smoked Salmon), 2 oz	0	0
Reuben Sandwich w/ ½ lb corned beef	28	1

DESSERTS

	C	F
Kipfel (Vanilla/Almd. Cookie), 1	7	0
New York Cheesecake, 1 slice	26	0
Pudding, 1 cup	48	0

MISCELLANEOUS

	C	F
Blintzes: Average, 1	25	
Blintzes: Average, w. Sour Crm. & Preserves	30	
Farfel, dry, ½ cup	21	
Gefilte Fish Balls: Reg., medium	4	
Gefilte Fish Balls: Reg., medium, w/Jellied Broth	6	
Gefilte Fish Balls: small / Cocktail size	2	0
Gefilte Fish Balls: Sweet, medium	4	0
Gefilte Fish Balls: Sweet, medium, w/ Jellied Broth	9	0
Kasha, ½ cup	20	
Knish / Cheese (Beiglach), 1	35	
Knish: Cheese, 1	35	
Knish: Kasha/Potato, 1	22	
Kreplach, beef, 1 piece	6	
Kugel, potato/noodle, 3" square	25	
Latkes (Potato Pancake), 4 3" pancakes	34	2
Lochshen: Plain, 1 cup	26	
Matzo Ball: 1 Extra large (3" diam)	24	
Matzo Ball: 1 large (2" diam)	12	
Matzo Balls: 2 small (1" diam)	12	
Matzo Farfel, 1 Cup	60	
Matzo Meal, 1 Cup	110	
Matzo: Average, full square	21	
Pierogi, potato/cheese, 1 piece	11	

Korean

	C	F
Bibimbab (Vege & Beef on Rice), 1 cup	89	3
Bulgogi (Barbecue Beef), 3.5 oz	15	0
Galbi (Short Ribs), 16 oz	16	0
Gujeolpan (Pancake w. Meat & Vegetables), 1 cup w/ 1 pancake	39	2
Japchae (Noodle w. Vege & Meat), 1¼ cups	34	2

	C	F
Kimchee (Cabbage Relish), ½ cup	6	0
Namool (Assorted Vegetables), 1 cup	9	1
Muguk (Radish & Chive Soup), 1 cup	6	0
Samgyetang (Ginseng Chicken Soup) w/ or w/o Chicken Skin, 1 cup	60	0
YukGaeJang (Spicy Beef Soup), 1¼ cups	5	0

Lebanese or Middle East

	C	F
Baba Ghannouj (Eggplant/Sesame Dip) 2 tbsp	2	0
Baklava, (Pastry, Nuts, Syrup), 1 pastry	18	1
Cabbage Rolls, (Cabbage Leaf, Meat, Rice), 1 roll	12	1
Couscous, (Semolina, Milk, Fruit, Nuts), 1 cup	43	2
Falafel (Chick Pea Fritter): Fried, 1 medium	4	1
Hummus, ¼ cup	5	1
Fried Kibbi, (Wheat, Meat, Pinenuts) 1 piece	15	1
Kafta, (Ground Lamb Saus. on Skewer), 1 skewer	2	0
Kibbeh Naye, (Raw Lamb, Bulgur & Spices) 1 cup	28	6
Lebanese Omelet (Egg, Spinach, Pinenuts, Onion), 4 oz	13	1
Pilaf (Rice, Onion, Raisins, Apr. Spice) 1 cup	60	2
Shawourma (Roast Beef), 4 oz	2	0
Shish Kabob, 1 stick	2	0
Spinach Pie, 3" piece	20	1
Sweet Almond Sanbusak (Pastry, Almonds, Spices), 1 piece	11	0
Tabouli, 4 oz	7	0
Tahini Sauce, 1 tbsp	2	0

Mexican

APPETIZERS

	C	F
Cheese Tostada, 6" round	15	0
Guacamole, 2 tbsp	2	0
Nachos w/beef & refried beans, 1½ cups	29	5

	C	F
Nachos w/cheese & jalapenos, 1 cup	17	0
Quesadilla, 9"	14	0
Refried Bean Dip, ½ cup	68	3
Salsa, 2 tbsp	2	0
Tortilla (corn), crisp, 6"	14	0
Tortilla (flour), soft, 6"	12	0

SOUPS, SALADS, SIDES

	C	F
Black Bean Soup, 1 cup	30	0
Corn Chips, 1 oz	15	1
Corn Gazpacho, 1 cup	25	1
Fried Bananas, 1 medium	22	1
Gazpacho w/Avocado, 1 cup	12	1
Mexican Cornbread, 4" square	54	1
Nopal Cactus Salad,	11	2
Papas Fritas (Fried Potatoes), ¾ cup	40	3
Pico De Gallo with Jicama, 1 cup	19	1
Pico De Gallo with Orange, 1½ cups	7	1
Refried Beans, 1 cup	40	3
Tomato Rice, 1¼ cups	50	1
Topopo Salad, 1 cup	18	3
Tortilla Chips, 1 oz	18	1

MAIN DISHES

	C	F
Burrito, Beef & Bean, average	22	3
Carne Asada, 9 oz	25	1
Carnitas, 6 oz	2	0
Chili con Carne: w. Beans, 1 cup	24	8
Chili con Carne: w/out Beans, 1 cup	10	0
Chili, plain, 1 cup	8	0
Chilis Rellenos Con Frijoles, ½ cup	9	1
Chimichanga (Beef), 5 oz	43	0
Chorizo Sausage, 2 oz	0	0
Costillas Ribs, 6 oz	0	0
Enchilada, average	49	2
Fajita, Chicken or Beef (Soft),	20	0
Flautas, 5-oz	35	1
Gorditas, 2	25	2

	C	F
Huevos Rancheros on Corn Tortillas, 2 cups	64	5
Mexican Omelet, 2 eggs	2	0
Shrimp in Chipolte Sauce, 1 cup	11	1
Sopes (Gorditas), 2 oz	27	2
Taco Salad w. Salsa,	85	5
Taco Sauce, average, ¼ cup	3	0
Taco, beef or chicken, 1	13	0
Tamales, Beef/Chicken, average	27	2
Taquitos, Beef & Cheese, average	36	3
Tortilla, Corn, 6" diam.	14	1
Tostada, beef or pork,	55	2

BEVERAGES

	C	F
Daiquiri (Banana), 1 cup	23	0
Daiquiri (Strawberry), 1 cup	40	1
Margarita, ½ cup	18	0
Pina Colada, 1 cup	15	0
Sangria, ½ cup	9	0

DESSERTS

	C	F
Banderilla (Pastry Puff), 1 shell	8	0
Bigotes, 7"	44	
Calvos, average	38	
Capirotada (Bread Pudding), 10 oz	107	3
Cinnamon Cookies, 2	13	0
Cocadas, 1 oz	15	0
Coconut Rice Pudding, ¾ cup	61	0
Concha (all colors), large (5" diam)	84	
Concha (all colors), medium (4" diam)	53	
Concha (all colors), small (3" diam)	38	
Cortadillo, 1 cookie	48	
Cream Puff with Custard, 4' ¼ oz	25	0
Cuerno, average	34	
Donus (Donuts), 4"	58	0
Elotes, average	51	
Empanadas, medium	42	3
Empanadas, small	28	2
Flan, ½ cup	26	0
Galletas Mixtas, 1 oz	16	
Guayaba, average	53	

	C	F
Jelly Rolls, average	46	0
Muffins/Nine Enbuelto, large	48	1
Orejas Ears, 3 oz	38	0
Pan Duke (Mexican Sweet Bread), 1 bun	45	
Panquecitos, average	36	
Piedras, average	76	
Polvorones, average	48	
Puerquitos, average	88	
Rebanadas, average	51	
Rice Pudding (Arroz Con Leche), ½ cup	24	0
Roles De Canela (Cin. Roll), average	81	
Roscas, average	44	
Semitas, average	46	
Sopapillas (flaky pastry puffs), 1 piece	10	0
Strawberry Creme Roll, average	45	1

Polish

	C	F
Cabbage Rolls w. Sour Cr., 2 small	30	0
Chicken Casserole w. Mushrooms, 1 cup	5	1
Kielbasa (Sausages, Onions, fried), 2 large	2	0
Meatballs in Sour Cream, 3 1½" balls	11	0
Pierogi, Fruit/Veg, 3"	15	1
Pork Goulash (Pork/Veg. Stew), 1½ cups	38	2
Pot Roast with Vegetables, 8 oz	28	2

Russian

SOUPS

	C	F
Borscht (beet soup), 1 cup	10	1
Cabbage Soup, 1 cup	2	0

MAIN DISHES

	C	F
Cabbage Rolls w/Lemon Sauce, 3 rolls	25	0
Chicken Kiev, 8 oz	9	0
Chicken Paprikash, 8 oz	12	0
Hungarian Goulash, 1 cup	3	0

	C	F
Pierogies, 1 cup	38	1
Steak Esterhazy, 8 oz	20	1

SIDE DISHES	CG	FG
Gefilte Fish, 2 balls	2	0
Kasha (Buckwheat Groats), ¾ cup	31	1
Kielbasa, 4 oz	2	0
Pickle (kosher, dill), large	3	1
Potato Pancakes, 4 3" pancakes	34	2
Salmon & Kasha, 5 oz	22	0

DESSERTS	CG	FG
Almond Kissel, average	57	1
Blintzes w/cottage cheese, 2 5" cakes	13	0
Rugelach, 5 small	33	0

Soul Foods

	CG	FG
Breakfast Sausage, fried, 2 patties	0	0
Brunswick Stew, 1 cup	19	1
Cornbread, homemade, 3" square	28	1
Fatback, raw	0	0
Ham Hock, 4 oz	2	0
Hog Maw, 4 oz	0	0
Hominy, cooked, ¾ cup	25	0
Hush Puppies, 5 pieces	35	1
Kale, cooked, ½ cup	4	1
Opossum, 4 oz	0	0
Oxtail, 4 oz	0	0
Pig Ear, ¼ ear	0	0
Pig Foot, ½ foot	0	0
Pig Tail, ⅓ tail	0	0
Poke Salad, cooked, ½ cup	3	0
Pork Brains, 4 oz	0	0
Pork Chitterlings, simmered, 3 oz	0	0
Pork Cracklings, ½ oz	0	0
Pork Neck Bones	0	0
Pork Skin, 1 cup	0	0
Pork Tongue, ⅓ tongue	0	0
Sousemeat, 4 oz	0	0
Succotash, ½ cup	17	3

	C	F
Sweet Potato Pie, ⅛ of 9" pie	45	2
Tripe, 2 oz	1	0
Vienna Sausage, 2 small	0	0

Spanish

SOUPS/APPETIZERS		
Gazpacho, 1 cup	12	1
Meat-Filled Turnovers, 2	6	0

MAIN DISHES		
Arroz Abanda (Fish with Rice), 1 cup	31	1
Arroz Con Pollo (Rice/Chicken Salad), 1 cup	32	1
Chicken Mole, 2 cups	14	1
Clams Marinara, 8 clams	22	0
Cochifrito (Lamb w. Lemon/ Garlic), average	5	0
Cochinillo Asado (Roast Suckling Pig), 2 slices	3	0
Cocido Madrileno (Madrid-Style Boiled Dinner), average	18	0
Fritadera de Ternera (Sauteed Veal), average	2	0
Green Pepper Sauteed, 1 pepper	6	1
Paella a la Valenciana (Chicken & Shellfish in Rice), 1½ cups	43	0
Pollo a la Espanola (Chicken), average	4	0
Ternera aljerez (Veal w. Sherry), average	6	0
Vegetable Stew, 1 cup	12	1
Zarzuela (Fish & Shellfish Medley), average serving	40	0

DESSERTS		
Bread Pudding, 1 cup	36	0
Flan deLeche (Caramel Custard), 1 cup	52	0
Pastry Puffs (Bunuelos), 4 small puffs	48	0

Thai

APPETIZERS		
Crab Rolls, 2	6	0
Dumplings (fried), 3	19	0

	C	F
Satay Pork, Beef or Chicken, 1 oz	0	0
Sauces: Peanut Satay, ½ cup	13	0
Spring Roll, 1 small	5	0

SOUPS/SALADS

	C	F
Green Papaya Salad, 1 cup	40	2
Lemon Grass Soup, 1 cup	3	0
Spicy Prawn Salad, 9 shrimp	15	0
Squid Salad, (¾ cup)	14	0
Thai Beef Salad, 1 cup	15	1
Thai Chicken Salad, 1 cup	17	1
Thai Noodle Salad, 1 cup	45	2
Tom Yam (Hot & Sour) Soup: Spicy Shrimp/Seafood, 1 cup	6	0
Vegetarian Soup, 1 cup	11	1

MAIN DISHES

	C	F
Chicken (w. veggies), Spicy stir-fry, 1 cup	14	2
Chicken in Peanut Sauce, 1¼ cups	14	1
Chicken with Lemon Grass, 8 oz	1	0
Coconut Shrimp (fried), 3 oz	23	1
Curry: Beef, 1 cup	8	1
Curry: Chicken w. Ginger, 1 cup	4	0
Curry: Pork, 1 cup	9	0
Curry: Thai Chicken, 1 cup	4	0
Fish with Lemon Grass, 6 oz	7	0
Pad Thai, large serving, 18 oz	125	5
Pork and Bamboo Shoots, ⅔ cup	4	1
Rice: Sticky Thai, Plain, 1 cup	36	0
Seafood Dip, 2 tbsp	1	0
Stir-fried Rice Noodles, 1 cup	40	2
Stir-fried Vegetables, 1 cup	18	2
Stuffed Eggplant, ½ eggplant	5	1
Thai Fried Noodles, 1½ cups	55	1
Tofu w. Vegetables, Spicy Garlic, stir-fry, 1 cup	18	1

DESSERTS

	C	F
Coconut Custard, ¾ cup	23	1
Mango with Sticky Rice, 1½ cups	80	1

Vietnamese

	C	F
Banh Cuon (Steam Rice w. Pork), 1 roll	8	0
Bo Nuong (Beef Satay), 2 sticks	4	0
Bo Xao Dau Phong (Ginger Beef w. Onion, Fish), average	10	0
Ca Chien Gung (Whole Snapper/Ging.), average	6	0
CanhChay (Veg/TofuSoup), 1 cup	13	1
Cari (Curry) Chicken, 1 cup	16	0
Cari (Curry) Chicken (1 cup), w. Rice Noodles (1 cup)	60	2
Cari (Curry) Chicken, (1 cup), w. Steamed Rice, (1 cup)	55	1
Cuu Xao Lan (Curried Lamb, Vegetables in Coconut), average	80	3
Ga Chien (Crisp Chicken w/ Plum Sauce), average serving	105	3
Ga Nuong (Chicken Satay & sauce), 4 oz	4	0
Ga Xao Rau (Marinated Chicken Braised w. Veg.), average	100	4
Gio Lua (Lean Pork Pie), ⅛ of pie	0	0
Goi Cuon (Cold Spring Rolls), each	7	0
ThitBoVien (Beef Balls), 6 pieces	2	0
Thit Heo Goi Baup Cai, (Spicy Cabbage Rolls w. Pork), 1 average	11	1
Soup Bun Bo Hue (Hot & Spicy) w or w/o Pork Feet, 1½ cups	35	0
Salad, Goi Du Du (Green Papaya Salad), average	29	3
Sauce: NuocCham (Hot Sauce)	1	0

FESTIVAL FOODS

SALADS

	C	F
Caesar Salad, 1 cup	15	1
Cole Slaw, 1 cup	37	2
Croutons, 2 tbsp	6	0
Egg Salad, ½ cup	7	0
Garden Salad (no dressing), 1 cup	6	1
Greek Salad, 2 cups	17	2
Macaroni Salad, ½ cup	13	1

	C	F
Pasta Salad, 1 cup	16	1
Potato Salad, 1 cup	35	4
Seafood Salad, ½ cup	10	0
Tuna Salad, ½ cup	7	0

SALTY SNACKS

	C	F
Nachos w. Cheese, 9" plate	70	4
Nachos w/Cheese, large order	132	7
Peanuts (in shell), 2 cups	24	3
Popcorn: Kettle Corn, large	220	24
Popcorn: Kettle Corn, small	110	12
Popcorn: Plain, large	96	24
Popcorn: Plain, small	48	12
Soft Pretzel, average twist pretzel	70	6

SIDE DISHES

	C	F
Artichoke: Fried, 9 pieces	24	9
Baked Beans, ½ cup	38	6
Baked Potato, large	100	10
Corn on the Cob, large ear	42	2
Curly Fries, 1½ cups	78	6
French Fries, 1½ cups	70	6
Garlic Bread, ¼ loaf	73	2
Egg Roll, fried, large	41	2
Mushrooms (Fried), 10–12 pieces	34	3
Onion Flower (Fried), 1 whole	140	2
Onion Rings, 3 large rings	40	0
Pickle, whole (6")	8	1
Pizza Bread (Pepperoni), ¼ loaf	76	2
Sweet Potato Strips (Fried), 4 pieces	106	5
Zucchini (Fried), 4 slices	42	6

ENTREES

	C	F
Bagel, large, approx 4" diameter	60	2
Beef Stew over Rice, 2 cups	61	1
Bratwurst/Sausage/ Kielbasa Sandwich	46	1
Burritos w. Bean/Beef, large	104	14
Chicken Nuggets, 6	26	1
Chicken Sandwich (breaded breast)	41	4
Chicken Strips, 4	33	1

	C	F
Chili, 1 cup	24	6
Corn dog, jumbo	36	2
Corn dog, regular	23	1
Falafel, large serving	85	18
Fried Rice: Beef, 6" bowl	136	4
Fried Rice: Chicken, 6" bowl	135	4
Gyros, 6"	42	2
Hamburger on bun, average	26	2
Hot Dog on bun, average	28	1
Hot Dog with Chili	32	3
Hot Dog, footlong on bun	41	1
Personal Pizza, 7"	80	5
Pizza, cheese or pepperoni, 1 slice	50	2
Ribs (Barbecued), ½ rack	21	0
Sandwich (Hoagie, Hero, Grinder, Sub), 8"	64	2
Roll (Kaiser), approx. 4" diameter	26	1
Shrimp (Fried), 10–12 pieces	36	1
Sloppy Joe, 1 medium	45	2
Spanakopita, 4" square	23	0
Taco (chicken or beef)	16	2
Tamale, medium	27	3
Taquitos, medium	36	4
Wraps/Roll-Up, large (15")	120	3
Wraps/Roll-Up, medium (10")	80	2
Wraps/Roll-Up, small (6")	48	1

SWEETS & DESSERTS

	C	F
Brownie (3.5" square)	44	
Candied Apple, large	80	3
Cheesecake on a Stick,	56	0
Chocolate Dipped Strawberry, 1 medium piece	15	0
Churros, medium	18	0
Cinnamon Roll, large	87	5
Cobbler, ¾ cup	62	2
Cotton Candy, medium bag	156	0
Cream Puff, medium	26	0
Dippin' Dots Ice Cream: small, ½ cup	17	0
Donut, Jumbo Twist	109	4

	C	F
Frozen Banana, choc covered	53	3
Frozen Yogurt in sugar cone	94	0
Fudge, 1½" square	25	0
Funnel Cake w/ Apple Cinnamon Topping	116	0
Funnel Cake w/ Cinn. & Sugar Topping	89	0
Funnel Cake w/ Strawberries & Cream Topping	96	0
Funnel Cake: Plain	80	0
Ice Cream: large, sugar cone, 14 oz	96	0
Ice Cream: small, sugar cone, 10 oz	83	0
Licorice (Rope), 24"	46	0
Oreos (Fried), 3 cookies	33	0
Pie Bar (Key Lime),	59	0
Puff-on-a-Stick, 4	44	0
Snickers (Fried)	42	2
Sno-Cone (w/syrup)	132	0
Strawberry Crepe, medium	36	1
Twinkie (Fried)	45	0
Twinkie Dog (Sundae)	89	0

BEVERAGES

	C	F
Beer (light), average 12 oz	5	0
Beer (nonalcoholic), average 12 oz	14	0
Beer (regular), average 12 oz	11	0
Drinks, Iced, 16 fl.oz	59	0
Frozen Lemonade, 1½ cups	78	0
Fruit Punch (sweetened), 8 oz	17	0
Hot Chocolate, 1 cup	25	0
Iced Tea (sweetened), 12 oz	38	0
Lemonade, 12 oz	24	0
Orange Julius, 2½ cups	96	0
Slushies, 2 cups	65	0
Smoothies: Berry Flavored, 2 cups	80	0
Soft Drink/Soda (diet), 12 oz	0	0
Soft Drink/Soda (sweetened), 12 oz	37	0

CONDIMENTS

	C	F
Barbecue Sauce, 1 tbsp	6	0
Buffalo Wing Sauce, 1 tbsp	2	0
Chili Sauce, 1 tbsp	4	0
Ketchup, 1 tbsp	4	0
Mayonnaise, 1 tbsp	1	0
Mustard, 1 tsp	0	0
Pickle (dill), 2 slices	0	0
Relish (sweet), 1 tbsp	5	0
Salad Dressing, 2 tbsp, average	2	0
Salsa, 2 tbsp	4	0

RESTAURANT & FAST FOOD

1 Potato 2®

	C	F
Fries, with Topping, average	82	0
Potato Skins, average, 1 (9 oz) serving	103	0
Potato, Gourmet or Lite, Baked, average, 1 serving	45	0
Potato, Ultra-Lites (Baked, no skin), average	48	0
Soups, average, 1 (13 oz) serving	81	0

7-11®

	CG	FG
Bakery Stix: Supreme, average, 1 (3.5 oz) serving	32	2
Big Eats: Smoked Turkey w/ Jack Cheese and Southwest Mayo, 1 (8.3 oz) serving	45	5
Breakfast Sandwich on Biscuit or Croissant, average, 1 sandwich	35	1
Breakfast Sandwich on Bun, average, 1 sandwich	23	11
Breakfast Sandwich on English Muffin, average, 1 (6 oz) serving	33	2
Burritos: Ramona, average, 1 burrito	40	0
Burritos: Reynolds, average, 1 (4.8 oz) serving	86	0

Applebee's®

MAIN ENTREES

	CG
Crispy Buttermilk Shrimp	83
Crispy Orange Skillet w. Noodles	209
Fiesta Lime Chkn w. Tortilla Strips	136

	C	F
Flour Tortilla (12")	52	
Grilled Shrimp Skewer	22	
Grilled Tilapia, w. Rice Pilaf & Mango Salsa	30	9
Low Fat Chicken Quesadilla	90	11
Low Fat Chicken Roma Roll-Up	83	6
Low Fat Garlic Chicken Pasta (full size portion)	134	3
Low Fat Talapia with Mango Salsa	54	6
Low Fat Veggie Quesadilla	86	11
Madeira Steak Tips w toast	82	
Mesquite Chicken Sandwich	42	
Oriental Chicken Salad Roll-Up	72	
Riblets w. sauce + fries	106	
Sizzling Chicken Skillet	43	10
Southwest Philly Roll-Up: w. Salsa	60	
Southwest Philly Roll-Up: w. Sour Cream	122	
Tango Chicken Sandwich	40	8
Teriyaki Steak and/or Shrimp Skewers	33	7
Tortilla Chicken Melt	50	6
Veggie Patch Pizza ⅙ of 10" pizza	12	

SOUPS & SALADS

	C	F
Onion au Gratin Soup	12	1
Grilled Citrus Chicken Salad		4
Grilled Shrimp Skewer Salad		7
Grilled Steak Caesar Salad: w. Toast	60	
Grilled Steak Caesar Salad: w/o Toast	44	
Low Fat Asian Chicken Salad (full size portion)	121	10
Low Fat Blackened Chicken Salad (full size portion)	42	5
Mesquite Chicken Salad	7	
Southwest Cobb Salad	13	

DESSERTS

	C	F
Berry Lemon Layer Cheesecake	34	2
Bikini Banana Low Fat Strawberry Shortcake	50	3
Blue Ribbon Brownie w. 2 scoops Ice Cream	105	

	C	F
Chocolate Raspberry Layer Cheesecake	46	3
Low Fat & Fabulous Brownie Sundae	72	4.6
Sizzling Apple Pie w. Ice Cream	146	
Triple Chocolate Meltdown Cake	107	

Arby's®

BREAKFAST

	C	F
Brkfst, Biscuit, Plain, Buttered or w/ meat, average, (1)	27	1
Brkfst, Croissant w/ Bacon, Ham or Sausage, average, (1)	29	1
Brkfst, French Toast w/syrup, (1)	32	0
Brkfst, French Toastix (no syrup), (1)	48	4
Brkfst, Sourdough w/ Bacon, Ham, or Sausage, average, (1)	67	3

ENTREES

	C	F
Chicken Finger 4-Pack, 1 serving	42	0
Chicken Finger Combo w/ Curly Fries, 1 serving	89	0
Chicken Finger Snack w/ Curly Fries, 1 serving	53	0
Light Grilled Chicken, 1 serving	30	3
Light Roast Chicken Deluxe, 1 serving	33	3
Light Roast Turkey Deluxe, 1 serving	33	3

SIDES

	C	F
Fries, Cheddar Curly, 1 serving	54	4
Fries, Curly, large, 1 serving	78	7
Fries, Curly, medium, 1 serving	50	4
Fries, Curly, small (3.7 oz), 1 serving	39	3
Fries, Homestyle, child size or side order, 1 serving	32	3
Fries, Homestyle, large, 1 serving	82	6
Fries, Homestyle, medium, 1 serving	55	4
Fries, Homestyle, small, 1 serving	44	3
Jalapeño Bites®, 1 order	30	2
Mozzarella Sticks, 1 order	34	2
Onion Petals, 1 order	43	2
Potato Cakes (2)	26	3
Potato, Baked Broccoli 'N Cheddar, (1)	51-71	7

	C	F
Potato, Baked Deluxe (10.4 oz) (1)	50	6
Potato, Baked with Butter & Sour Cream, (1)	48-65	6

DRESSINGS, CONDIMENTS & EXTRAS

	C	F
Condiment, German Mustard Packet, 1 serving	0	0
Condiments, Ketchup Packet, 1 serving	2	0
Condiments, Mayonnaise Packet (2 tsp),	11	0
Condiments, Mayonnaise Packet, Light, Cholesterol Free, 1 serving	1	0
Croutons, Cheese & Garlic, 1 serving	10	0
Croutons, Seasoned, 1 serving	5	1
Dressing, Asian Sesame, 1.9 oz	14	
Dressing, BBQ Vinaigrette, 1 serving	14	
Dressing, Bleu Cheese, 1 serving	3	0
Dressing, Buttermilk Ranch, 2 oz	13	1
Dressing, Buttermilk Ranch, Reduced Calorie, 2 oz	2	0
Dressing, Caesar, 1 serving	1	0
Dressing, Honey French, 1 serving	18	<1
Dressing, Italian Parmesan, 1 serving	4	0
Dressing, Italian, Fat Free (Reduced Calorie), 2 oz	3	<1
Dressing, Light Balsamic Vinaigrette, 2 oz	13	
Dressing, Thousand Island, 1 serving	9	0

SALADS

	C	F
Chicken Club w/ or w/o Buttermilk dressing, average, 1 serving	34	
Chicken Finger (dressing not included), 1 serving	39	3
Garden Regular or Side, average, 1 serving	14	6
Grilled Chicken, 1 serving	14	6
Salad, Grilled Chicken Caesar (dressing not incl.), 1 serving	8	3
Martha's Vineyard w/ Raspberry Vinaigrette & Almonds, 1 serving	40	5
Martha's Vineyard w/o Raspberry Vinaigrette & Almonds, 1 serving	23	4
Roast Chicken, 1 serving	15	6

	C	F
Santa Fe w/ Santa Fe Dressing & Tortilla Strips, 1 serving	53-62	5.5
Santa Fe w/o Dressing & Tortilla Strips, 1 serving	29-40	5
Side, 1 serving	7	2
Turkey Club (dressing not included), 1 serving	9	3

SANDWICHES

	C	F
Arby's Melt With Cheddar, (1)	36	2
Arby-Q®, (1)	40	2
Beef 'N Cheddar, (1)	43	2
Big Montana®, (1)	41	3
Chicken Bacon 'N Swiss, (1)	49	2
Chicken Breast Fillet, (1)	47	2
Chicken Cordon Bleu, (1)	47	2
Chicken Salad, Market Fresh®, (1)	78	6
French Dip, (1)	42	2
French Dip & Swiss, (1)	51	3
Giant Roast Beef, (1)	41	3
Grilled Chicken Deluxe, (1)	37	2
Hot Ham 'N Swiss, (1)	35	1
Junior Roast Beef, (1)	34	2
Philly Beef Supreme, (1)	59	3
Regular Roast Beef, (1)	34	2
Roast Beef, (1)	47	3
Roast Beef & Swiss, Market Fresh, (1)	73	5
Roast Chicken Caesar, Market Fresh, (1)	75	5
Roast Chicken Club, (1)	38	2
Roast Ham & Swiss, Market Fresh, (1)	74	5
Roast Turkey & Swiss, Market Fresh, (1)	75	5
Sub, Hot Ham 'N Swiss, (1)	45	3
Sub, Italian, (1)	49	3
Sub, Philly Beef 'N Swiss, (1)	46	4
Sub, Turkey, (1)	51	2
Super Roast Beef, (1)	47	3

SANDWICHES (LOW CARBYS®)

	C	F
Regular Roast Beef, (1)	1	0
Roast Beef & Swiss, (1)	3	1

	C	F
Roast Ham & Swiss, (1)	5	0
Roast Turkey & Swiss, (1)	4	0
Roast Turkey, Ranch & Bacon, (1)	5	0
Super Roast Beef, (1)	2	1
Ultimate BLT, (1)	6	6

WRAPS

	C	F
Chicken Caesar Market Fresh® Low Carbys, 1 each	46	
Chicken Cheddar Jack, 1 each	59	
Chicken Salad, 1 each	52	
Roast Turkey, Ranch & Bacon Market Fresh® Low Carbys, 1 each	48	
Southwest Chicken Market Fresh® Low Carbys,	45	
Ultimate BLT Market Fresh® Low Carbys,	48	

SAUCES

	C	F
Au Jus, 1 serving	1	0
Arby's® Packet (0.5 ounce),	4	0
BBQ Dipping (1 ounce),	10	0
Bronco Berry®, 1 serving	23	0
Honey Mustard (1 ounce),	5	0
Horsey® Packet, 1 serving	3	0
Marinara, 1 serving	4	0
Tangy Southwest®, 1 serving	3	0

BEVERAGES

	C	F
Milk Shake, Vanilla, Choc., Strawberry, or Jamocha, average, regular (13.2 oz) Size	84	0
Milk Shake, Vanilla, Choc., Strawberry, or Jamocha, average, large Size	110	0

DESSERTS

	C	F
Apple Turnover (Iced), 1 each	65	2
Cherry Turnover (Iced), 1 each	63	1
Gourmet Chocolate Cookie, 1 each	26	

Atlanta Bread Company®

BAGELS & BREADS

	C	F
Bagels, All except Low Carb, average (1)	73	3

	C	F
Bagels, Low Carb, Cranberry Walnut (1)	65	
Breads: ABC Roll, 1 roll	54	
Breads: Per Thick Slice Asiago, (1)	29	1
Breads: Per Thick Slice Asiago Strip, (1)	28	
Breads: Per Thick Slice Challah, (1)	29	0.5
Breads: Per Thick Slice Cinnamon Raisin Loaf, (1)	30	2
Breads: Per Thick Slice Cracked Wheat, (1)	30	2

SANDWICHES (NO CHEESE OR DRESSING)

	C	F
ABC Special on French Roll, (1)	64	2
Peanut Butter & Jelly, (1)	99	
Roasted Turkey Breast, (1)	61	2
Tangy Roast Beef, (1)	59	2
Tuna, 4 oz, (1)	30	1
Veggie on Nine Grain, (1)	63	2

FOCACCIA

	C	F
Bella Basil on Tom. & Rosemary, (1)	58	
California Avocado on Tom. On., (1)	71	7
Chicken Salad, 4 oz, (1)	2	1
Grilled Cheese on French Bread, (1)	57	
Honey Maple Ham, (1)	63	2
Hot Pastrami, (1)	59	2

PANINIIS

	C	F
Chicken Pesto, (1)	78	4
Cordon Bleu, (1)	76	3
Cuban Pork Loin, (1)	82	4
Italian Vegetarian, (1)	81	5
Turkey Club, (1)	79	3

SALADS

	C	F
Caesar, (1)	9	2
Chicken Salad on Lettuce, (1)	4	0
Chopstix Chicken, (1)	38	6
Extra Croutons, 0.5 oz, (1)	6	
Fruit, 10 oz, (1)	34	2
Greek, (1)	13	2
House, (1)	9	2

	C	F
Tuna Salad on Lettuce, (1)	4	
Add Grilled Chicken, 2.5 oz, (1)	2	

SOUPS

	C	F
Black Bean & Ham, 10 oz	40	
Chicken Tortilla, 10 oz	20	
Chunky Baked Potato, 10 oz	30	
Classic Chicken Noodle, 10 oz	21	
Cream of Broccoli, 10 oz	19	
Creamy Tomato, 10 oz	10	
French Onion w. Toppings, 10 oz	16	
Garden Vegetable, 10 oz	19	
Homestyle Chicken'n Dumpling, 10 oz	25	
New England Clam Chowder, 10 oz	24	
Pasta Fagioli, 10 oz	24	
Spicy Chicken Gumbo, 10 oz	16	
Wisconsin Cheese, 10 oz	21	

MUFFIN TOPS

	C	F
Banana Nut, (1)	39	
Blueberry, (1)	31	
Chocolate Chip, (1)	52	
Mocha, (1)	53	
Pumpkin, (1)	54	

Au Bon Pain®

BREADS, BAGELS AND SPREADS

	C	F
Bagel, Dutch Apple, (1)	99	
Bagel, French Toast or Cinnamon Raisin, average, (1)	74	
Bagel, Plain or Asiago Cheese, average, (1)	60	
Breads, Braided Plain Roll (1)	62	
Breads, Bread Bowl (1)	127	
Breads, Bread Rolls: Hearth (1)	44	
Breads, Foccacia (1)	58	
Breads, Four Grain Bread, 1 slice	58	
Breads, Rosemary Garlic Breadstick, 1 stick	33	
Spreads: Plain Cream Cheese, 2 oz	4	
Spreads: Smoked Salmon, 2 oz	3	
Spreads: Sun Dried Tomato, Veggie, 2 oz	3	

SANDWICHES & WRAPS

	C	F
Asian Chicken Salad Sandwich, (1)	50	
Breakfast Sandwich on Bagel Plain or w/ w/o meat (1)	63	
Chicken & Mozzarella Foccacia (1)	73	
Chicken Caesar Wrap (1)	63	
Chicken Tarragon w. Field Onions Sandwich, (1)	71	
Fields & Feta Wrap (1)	90	
Fresh Mozzarella, Tomato w. Pesto Sandwich, (1)	67	
Grilled Chicken w. Blue Cheese Sandwich, (1)	64	
Mediterranean Wrap (1)	80	
Roasted Turkey Cranberry Sandwich, (1)	80	
Southwestern Tuna Wrap (1)	68	
Spicy Tuna on Multigrain Sandwich, (1)	72	
Tuna w. Cheddar & Peppers Sandwich, (1)	62	
Turkey w. Guacamole & Swiss Sandwich, (1)	77	

SOUPS & SALADS

	C	F
Fruit Cup: large, 12 oz	32	
Fruit Cup: small, 6 oz	16	
Salad, Caesar Salad, (1)	23	
Salad, Chefs Salad (1)	8	
Salad, Garden Salad (1)	10	
Salad, Gorgonzola& Walnut (1)	10	
Salad, Mediterranean Chicken (1)	14	
Salad, Thai Chicken (1)	14	
Salad, Tuna Garden (1)	25	
Salad, Tuna Nicoise (1)	19	
Salad, Turkey Medallion Cobb (1)	27	
Soups, Broccoli Cheddar, 8 oz	13	
Soups, Chicken Noodle, 8 oz	11	
Soups, Corn Chowder, 8 oz	25	
Soups, Garden Vegetable, 8 oz	7	
Soups, Split Pea w. Ham, 8 oz	23	
Soups, Vegetarian Chili, 8 oz	30	
Yogurt & Fruit, average, 15 oz	75	

MUFFINS & CROISSANTS	C	F
Croissants, Chocolate, (1)	61	
Croissants, Filled: Plain, (1)	44	
Croissants, Ham & Cheese, (1)	46	
Croissants, Raspberry, (1)	55	
Croissants, Spinach & Cheese, (1)	32	
Croissants, Sweet Cheese, (1)	52	
Muffins, Blueberry, (1)	76	
Muffins, Chocolate, (1)	83	
Muffins, Corn Chunk, (1)	64	
Muffins, Cranberry Walnut, (1)	69	
Muffins, Low Fat: Chocolate Cake, (1)	74	
Muffins, Raisin Bran, (1)	100	
Muffins, Triple Berry, (1)	61	

BEVERAGES	C	F
Cappuccino, 16 fl.oz	12	
Frozen Mocha Blast, 16 fl.oz	57	
Iced Tea, 22 fl. oz	30	
Mocha Blast, 16 fl.oz	54	

DESSERTS	C	F
Brownie: Blonde w. nuts, (1)	57	
Brownie: Chocolate Chip w. nuts, (1)	61	
Cakes & Bars, Apple Strudel, 1 piece	56	
Cakes & Bars, Cherry Strudel, 1 piece	49	
Cakes & Bars, Cinnamon Roll, 1 piece	67	
Cakes & Bars, Pecan Brownie, 1 piece	55	
Cookies, Chocolate Chip, (1)	41	
Cookies, English Toffee, (1)	26	
Cookies, Oatmeal Raisin, (1)	42	
Cookies, Shortbread, (1)	35	

Auntie Anne's®

PRETZELS	C	F
Almond or Whole wheat w/ or w/o butter, 1 pretzel	72	
Cinnamon Sugar w/ butter, 1 pretzel	83	
Cinnamon Sugar w/o butter, 1 pretzel	74	
Garlic or Sour Cream & Onion w/ or w/o butter, 1 pretzel	67	
Glazin' Raisin® w/ or w/o butter, 1 pretzel	106	

	C	F
Jalapeño w/ or w/o butter, 1 pretzel	58	
Original w/ or w/o butter, 1 pretzel	72	
Parmesan Herb w/ or w/o butter, 1 pretzel	72	
Sesame w/ or w/o butter, 1 pretzel	63	
Stix, 4 sticks w/ or w/o butter, 1 pretzel	48	

EXTRAS	C	F
Caramel Dip, 1.5 oz	27	
Cheese Sauce; Hot Salsa Cheese, average	4	
Chocolate Flavored Dip, 1.25 oz	24	
Light Cream Cheese, 1.25 oz	1	
Marinara Sauce, 1.25 oz	4	
Strawberry Cream Cheese, 1.25 oz	4	
Sweet Mustard, 1.25 oz	8	

BEVERAGES	C	F
Auntie Anne's Lemonade, 22 fl.oz	43	
Dutch Ice, Blue Raspberry, 20 fl. oz	55	
Dutch Ice, Kiwi-Banana, 20 fl. oz	63	
Dutch Ice, Lemonade, 20 fl. oz	110	
Dutch Ice, Mocha, 20 fl. oz	105	
Dutch Ice, Orange Creme, 20 fl. oz	92	
Dutch Ice, Pina Colada, Strawberry, 20 fl. oz	125	
Dutch Ice, Wild Cherry, 20 fl oz	69	
Dutch Smoothie, Blue Raspberry, 20 fl oz	65	
Dutch Smoothie, Kiwi-Banana, 20 fl oz	68	
Dutch Smoothie, Lemonade, 20 fl oz	95	
Dutch Smoothie, Mocha, 20 fl oz	90	
Dutch Smoothie, Orange Creme, 20 fl oz	83	
Dutch Smoothie, Pina Colada, 20 fl oz	79	
Dutch Smoothie, Strawberry, Wild Cherry, 20 fl oz	74	

Baja Fresh®

MAIN ENTREES	C	F
Burrito, Baja, w. Charbroiled Chicken or Steak incl. cheese, (1)	75	11
Burrito, Bare w. Charbroiled Chicken incl. cheese, (1)	99	22
Burrito, Bare, Vegetarian incl. cheese, (1)	172	32
Burrito, Bean & Cheese w. Chicken. Charbroiled Steak or Vegetarian, incl. cheese, (1)	177	30
Burrito, Dos Manos: w. Chicken or Charbroiled Steak incl. cheese, (1)	101	14
Burrito, Mexicano: w. Chicken or Charbroiled Steak incl. cheese, (1)	124	20
Burrito, Ultimo: w. Charbroiled Chicken or Steak incl. cheese, (1)	90	10
Burrito, Grilled Vegetarian, (1)	100	16
Burrito, Fajita w. Chicken or Steak, (1)	88	
Burrito, Enchilado Style: (add to any Dos Manos), (1)	44	
Fajitas, Charbroiled Chicken or Steak w. Corn Tortillas, (1)	164	33
Nachos: w. Charbroiled Steak, Cheese or Chicken, average, (1)	166	33
Quesadilla: w. Chicken, Charbroiled Steak, or Cheese & Chips, (1)	80	10
Quesadilla: Vegetarian w. Chips, (1)	92	12
Taco, Baja Fish (Breaded), (1)	31	
Taco, Baja Mahi Mahi, (1)	32	6
Taco, Baja Style Taco w. Charbroiled Chicken, Steak or Wild Gulf Shrimp, (1)	25	

SALADS		
Baja Ensalada: No Dressing, w. Charbroiled Chicken or Steak, (1)	18	
Baja Ensalada: No Dressing, w. Charbroiled Fish, (1)	27	
Chile Lime Chicken, (1)	75	
Chipotle Glaze Charbroiled Chicken, (1)	56	
Ensalada w. Charbroiled Mahi Mahi, (1)	27	

	C	F
Taquitos: w. Chicken or Steak, Beans or Rice, (1)	68	

Baskin Robbins®

Chocolate, Reg. Scoop	31	0
Vanilla, Reg. Scoop	24	0
Chocolate Chip, Reg. Scoop	26	0
Pralines 'n Cream, Reg. Scoop	33	0
Jamoca Almond Fudge, Reg. Scoop	30	0
Rainbow Sherbet, Reg. Scoop	34	0
Daiquiri Ice, Reg. Scoop	33	0
Peachy Keen Sorbet, Reg. Scoop	29	0
Espresso 'n Cream Low Fat, Reg. Scoop	31	0
Maui Brownie Madness Low Fat Yogurt, Reg. Scoop	38	0
Thin Mint w/ NutraSweet, Reg. Scoop	27	0
Peach Crumb Pie w/ NutraSweet, Reg. Scoop	27	0
Chocolate Soft Serve Nonfat Yogurt w/ nutrasweet, 5 oz	39	0
Café Mocha Soft Serve Yogurt w/ NutraSweet, small	27	0
Chocolate Ice Cream Shake, Regular Size	80	0
Vanilla Ice Cream Shake, regular size	69	0
Cappuccino Blast w/ Whipped Cream, regular Size	44	0
Very Strawberry Smoothie w/ Soft Serve Ice Cream, regular Size	70	0

Ben & Jerry's®

BODY & SOUL		
Body & Soul: Cherry Garcia, ½ cup	22	2
Body & Soul: Chocolate Chip Cookie Dough, ½ cup	26	1
Body & Soul: Chocolate Fudge Brownie, ½ cup	25	2
Body & Soul: Half Baked, ½ cup	29	2

FROZEN YOGURT	C	F
Frozen Yogurt: Cherry Garcia, ½ cup	32	<1
Frozen Yogurt: Chocolate Fudge Brownie or Half Baked, ½ cup	35	<1
Frozen Yogurt: Low Fat: Black Raspberry, ½ cup	28	
Frozen Yogurt: Phish Food, ½ cup	41	1
Frozen Yogurt: Vanilla, ½ cup	25	

ORIGINAL FLAVORS

	C	F
Original Brownie Batter, Choc. Chip Cookie Dough, Choc. Fudge Original Brownie, 1 pint	32	
Original Butter Pecan, 1 pint	20	
Original Cherry Garcia, Mint Chocolate Cookie, Strawberry, 1 pint	26	
Original Chocolate, 1 pint	25	
Original Chubby Hubby, Coffee, Pistachio or Vanilla, 1 pint	21	
Original Chunky Monkey, Everything But The . . . , NY Super Fudge Chunk, 1 pint	30	
Original Coffee Heath Bar Crunch, Primary Berry Graham, Vanilla Heath Bar Crunch, Vanilla Swiss Original Almond, 1 pint	29	
Original Fudge Central, Oatmeal Cookie Chunk, 1 pint	31	
Original Half Baked, 1 pint	34	
Original Karamel Sutra, 1 pint	33	
Original Peanut Butter Cup, Uncanny Cashew, 1 pint	27	
Original Phish Food, 1 pint	37	

NOVELTIES

	C	F
Peace Pops: Cherry Garcia, (1)	29	
Peace Pops: Cookie Dough, (1)	41	
Peace Pops: One Sweet Whirled, (1)	28	
Peace Pops: Vanilla, (1)	26	
Peace Pops: Vanilla with Heath Toffee, (1)	30	
Witch Cookie Switch, (1)	45	

SINGLE SERVING SIZE

	C	F
Single Size Cherry Garcia, 1 single size	22	
Single Size Chocolate Fudge Brownie, 1 single size	28	
Single Size Cookie Dough, 1 single size	26	
Single Size Vanilla, 1 single size	17	

SORBET

	C	F
Sorbet: average all flavors, ½ cup	27	2

Big Apple Bagels®

BAGELS

	C	F
All types, average, 5 oz	72	
My Favorite Muffin: Honey Grain, 4 oz	61	
My Favorite Muffin: Other varieties, 4 oz	66	

MUFFINS

	C	F
My Favorite Muffin: Blueberry, Jumbo	66	
My Favorite Muffin: Blueberry, Fat Free, Jumbo	78	
My Favorite Muffin: Chocolate Chip, Jumbo	81	
My Favorite Muffin: Chocolate, Fat Free, Jumbo	84	

SPREADS

	C	F
Cream Cheese: Plain, 2 tbsp	2	
Cream Cheese: Honey Cinnamon; Very Berry, 2 tbsp	3	
Cream Cheese: Lite varieties, average, 2 tbsp	2	

SOUPS

	C	F
Boston Clam/Potato Chowder, 8 fl oz	20	
Chicken Noodle; Beef Pot Roast, 8 fl oz	12	
Garden Vegetable, 8 fl oz	22	
Minestrone, 8 fl oz	26	
Split Pea w. Ham; Hearty Vegetable, 8 fl oz	16	

Blimpie®

SANDWICHES

	C	F
Sub, Cold: Blimpie Best on white w/cheese, 6"	51	

	C	F
Sub, Cold: Club on white w/cheese, 6"	50	
Sub, Cold: Ham & Swiss Cheese on white, 6"	51	
Sub, Cold: Roast Beef on white w/cheese, 6"	49	
Sub, Cold: Seafood, on white, no Cheese, 6"	58	
Sub, Cold: Tuna on white w/cheese, 6"	51	
Sub, Cold: Turkey on white w/cheese, 6"	49	
Paninis: Cuban, (1)	50	
Paninis: Grilled Chicken Caesar, (1)	50	
Paninis: Turkey Italiano, (1)	44	
Wraps: Chicken Caesar, (1)	56	
Wraps: Zesty Italian, (1)	74	
Sub, Hot: Grilled Chicken on White, 6"	50	
Sub, Hot: Meatball w. Cheese on White, 6"	55	
Sub, Hot: Mexi Max on White, 6"	65	
Sub, Hot: Steak & Onion Melt w. Cheese on White, 6"	49	
Sub, Hot: VegiMax on White, 6"	60	

SALADS AND DRESSINGS

	C	F
Salads: Chef Salad, (1)	9	
Salads: Grilled Chicken, (1)	9	
Salads: Seafood Salad, (1)	15	
Salads: Tuna, (1)	8	
Dressings & Sauces: Caesar, (1)	5	
Dressings & Sauces: Blimpie, 1.5 oz	24	

SOUPS

	C	F
Chicken w. White & Wild Rice, ½ cup	21	
Garden Vegetable	14	
Home-style Chicken Noodle, ½ cup	18	
Vegetable Beef, ½ cup	13	

DESSERTS

	C	F
Cookies: Oatmeal Raisin, 1 cookie	27	
Cookies: Sugar, 1 cookie	24	

	C	F
Cookies: Other varieties, average, 1 cookie	26	

Bob Evans®

BREAKFAST	C	F
Belgian Waffle, (1)	57	2
Brkfst. Combinations: Country Biscuit, (1)	51	1
Brkfst. Combinations: Fruit & Yogurt Plate, 1 serving	92	8
Brkfst. Combinations: Home Fries, 1 serving	28	
Brkfst. Combinations: Lite Sausage Breakfast, 1 serving	48	4
Brkfst. Combinations: Pot Roast Hash Breakfast, 1 serving	35	4
Brkfst. Combinations: Sirloin Steak, 1 serving	3	
Crepes Combos: Raspberry, (2)	58	5
Crepes Combos: Strawberry Banana, (2)	56	4
Crepes, Plain, (1)	14	0
Farm Fresh Eggs: Fresh Eggs Benedict, 1 serving	35	2
Farm Fresh Eggs: Hardboiled Egg Beaters, 1.5 serving	1	
Farm Fresh Eggs: Over Easy (1), 1 serving	1	
Farm Fresh Eggs: Scrambled (1), 1 serving	3	0
Farm Fresh Eggs: Scrambled Egg Beaters, 1 serving	2	
French Toast, Stuffed, 10 oz	58	3
Fruit Cup, 1 serving	38	4
Grits, 1 serving	28	2
Hotcakes: Multigrain, (1)	43	3
Hotcakes: Blueberry, (1)	47	2
Hotcakes: Buttermilk, (1)	43	1
Hotcakes: Cinnamon, (1)	56	1
Mush, 1 slice	14	1
Oatmeal, plain, 1 bowl	32	4
Omelettes: Cheese or Three Cheese, w/ or w/o Egg Beaters, average, 2 serving	4	1

	C	F
Omelettes: Farmer's Market, w/ or w/o Egg Beaters, average, 2 serving	16	3
Omelettes: Ham and Cheese, w/ or w/o Egg Beaters, average, 2 serving	5	1
Omelettes: Sausage & Cheese, 2 serving	47	3
Omelettes: Sausage & Cheese, Egg Beaters, 3 serving	54	5
Omelettes: Southwestern Chicken, 1 serving	5	
Omelettes: Turkey Florentine, w/ or w/o Egg Beaters, average, 3 serving	7	2
Omelettes: Western, w/ or w/o Egg Beaters, average,	10	2
Omelettes: Border Scramble, w/ or w/o Egg Beaters, average, 2 serving	15	3
Sausage & Cheese Breakfast Bake, 9.6 oz	11	1
Sausage Breakfast Burger, 7.4 oz	32	1
Sausage Sandwich, Double, (1)	31	1
Sirloin Steak, 4.9 oz	3	0
Strawberry Yogurt, 5 oz	28	1
Sunshine Skillet, 17.4	48	4

MAIN ENTREES

	C	F
Chicken Pot Pie, 1 serving	46	
Chicken-n-Noodles, 1 serving	32	
Country Fried Steak w/ Gravy, 1 serving	31	
Country Fried Steak w/o Gravy, 1 serving	26	
Fried Chicken (1), 1 serving	9	
Fried Shrimp, 1 serving	8	
Grilled Chicken (1), 1 serving	0	
Lunch Savors: Chicken & Broccoli Alfredo Pasta, 1 serving	49	
Lunch Savors: Quesadillas: Chicken, 1 serving	50	
Lunch Savors: Stir-Fry: Grilled Chicken, 1 serving	55	

	C	F
Lunch Savors: Stir-Fry: Grilled Shrimp, 1 serving	60	
Lunch Savors: Stir-Fry: Vegetable, 1 serving	55	
Meat Loaf (Beef & Pork), 1 serving	14	
Salmon, 1 serving	12	

KIDS MENU

	C	F
Hot Diggety Dog w/ Bun, plain, 1 serving	23	
Mini Cheeseburgers, 1 serving	20	
Pizza Pizzazz, 1 serving	57	
Plenty-O-Pancakes, 1 serving	79	
Quesadilla, Chicken, 1 serving	39	
Spaghetti & Meatballs, 1 serving	57	
Turkey Lurkey, 1 serving	1	
Mac & Cheese, 1 serving	45	

SALADS

	C	F
Chicken Salad, (1)	77	
Cobb w/ Grilled Chicken, average, (1)	11	
Country Spinach, average, (1)	12	
Frisco w/ Grilled Chicken, (1)	9	
Frisco: w/ Fried Chicken, (1)	26	
Wildfire Chicken w/ Fried Chicken, (1)	74	
Wildfire Chicken w/ Grilled Chicken, (1)	57	

SANDWICHES & BURGERS

	C	F
Bacon Cheeseburger, (1)	31	
Big BLT, (1)	29	
Bob's BLT & E, (1)	48	
Cheeseburger, (1)	31	
Fried Chicken Club, (1)	40	
Grilled Chicken Club, (1)	32	
Grilled Chicken, (1)	30	
Hamburger, (1)	30	
Pot Roast, (1)	62	
Turkey Bacon Melt, (1)	56	

SIDES	C	F
Bacon, 1 strip	0	0
Baked Potato Seasoned, Loaded, (1)	57	
Baked Potato Seasoned, Plain, (1)	54	
Canadian Bacon, 1 slice	0	0
Cheddar Broccoli Florets, 1 serving	14	
Coleslaw, 4 oz	18	
Corn, Buttered Sweet, 4.5 oz	18	
Garden Side Salad, 5.3 oz	26	
Home Fries, 5 oz	28	3
Lite Sausage Link, 1 link	0	0
Mashed Potatoes, 5 oz	15	
Mushrooms, Grilled, 7.9 oz	10	
Onion Rings, 6 oz	49	
Rice Pilaf, 5 oz	32	
Sausage Link, 2 links	0	0
Sausage Patty, 1 patty	0	0
Sausage Sandwich Patty, 2.7 oz	0	0
Smoked Ham, 1 slice	2	0

SPECIALTY BREADS

	C	F
Banana Nut, 1 slice	30	
Cinnamon Swirl Roll, Frosted, 1 roll	76	
Dinner Roll, 1 roll	34	
English Muffin, 1 muffin	28	
Garlic Bread, 2 oz	16	
Sourdough, 1.7 oz	26	
Texas Toast, 8 oz	12	

BEVERAGES

	C	F
Iced Tea: Blackberry	23	
Iced Tea: Raspberry; Strawberry	20	
Iced Tea: regular, Unsweetened	1	

DESSERTS

	C	F
Pies: Apple Dumpling A La Mode, 1 serving	119	
Pies: Apple Dumpling, 1 serving	100	
Pies: Banana Cream, 1 serving	52	
Pies: Coconut Cream, 1 serving	57	
Pies: Hershey's Hot Fudge Cake, 1 serving	94	
Pies: Lemon Meringue, 1 serving	89	

	C	F
Pies: Oreo Cheesecake, 1 serving	61	
Pies: Pumpkin, 1 serving	69	
Sundae: Fudge, 1 serving	78	
Sundae: Reese's, 1 serving	104	

Boston Market®

ENTREES

	C	F
Crispy-Baked Country Chicken w. Gravy, 1 serving	33	
Double-Sauced Angus: Meatloaf, 1 serving	22	
Meatloaf & Beef Gravy, 1 serving	27	
Half Sweet Garlic Rotisserie Chicken w. skin, ½ whole chicken, 1 serving	4	
Hand-Carved: Honey Glazed Ham, 5 oz, 1 serving	10	0
Rotisserie Turkey, 1 serving	3	
Pastry Top Chicken Pot Pie, 1 serving	57	
¼ Chicken: White meat w. skin / wing, 5.3 oz, 1 serving	2	0
¼ Chicken: White meat w/o skin or wing, 4.9 oz, 1 serving	2	0
¼ Chicken: Dark meat w. skin, 4.4 oz, 1 serving	2	0
¼ Chicken: Dark meat w/o skin, 5.3 oz, 1 serving	1	0

HOT SIDE DISHES

	C	F
Butternut Squash, 1 serving	25	6
Creamed Spinach, 6.4 oz, ¾ cup	11	2
Mashed Potatoes w. Gravy, 7.1 oz, ¾ cup	32	3
Cinnamon Apples, 6.4 oz, ¼ cup	56	3
Macaroni & Cheese, 6.8 oz, ¾ cup	33	1
Steamed Vegetable Medley, 3.6 oz, 1 serving	6	2
Sweet Corn, 1 serving	30	

SALADS

	C	F
Caesar Side, 1 salad	13	0.5
Rotisserie Chicken Caesar, 1 salad	19	
Southwest Chicken, 1 salad	40	

SANDWICHES & BURGERS	C	F
Chicken Carver w. Cheese & Sauce, 10.7 oz, 1 sandwich	64	4
Meatloaf Carver w. Cheese, 13.2 oz, 1 sandwich	93	5
Turkey Carver w. Cheese & Sauce, 10.7 oz, 1 sandwich	66	4

SOUPS	C	F
Hearty Chicken Noodle Soup, 6.7 oz, 6.7 oz	8	0
Tortilla Soup w. toppings, 6.5 oz, 6.5 oz	18	2
Tortilla Soup w. w/o toppings, 5.5 oz, 5.5 oz	7	1

DESSERTS	C	F
Apple Pie 5.5 oz, 1 slice	73	3
Caramel Pecan Brownie, 1 brownie	144	
Chocolate Brownie 5 oz, 1 brownie	88	6
Chocolate Cake 5.6 oz, 1 slice	86	2
Chocolate Mania, 1 serving	37	
Cornbread 2.4 oz, 1 serving	27	1
Family Size: Apple Pie, 1 pie	54	
Family Size: Caramel Pecan Brownie, 1 brownie	22	
Family Size: Chocolate Brownie, 1 brownie	22	
Molten Fudge Cake, 1 slice	34	
Nestle Toll House Cookie, average 3 oz, 1 cookie	51	2
Strawberry Bliss, 1 serving	16	

Bruegger's Bagels®

	C	F
Bagels: Plain/Salt/Sesame/Garlic, 1	68	4
Bagels: Blueberry/Cranb. Or./Cinn. Raisin, 1	68	4
Bagels: Chocolate Chip, 1	69	4
Bagels: Everything/Onion/Sundried Tom., 1	65	4
Cream Cheese: average, 2 oz	8	0
Cream Cheese: Light varieties, average, 2 oz	6	0
Hummus, 2 oz	8	2

	C	F
Breakfast Sandwiches: Egg & Cheese, 1	66	4
Breakfast Sandwiches: Egg & Cheese & Bacon, 1	66	4
Breakfast Sandwiches: Egg & Cheese& Ham, 1	66	4
Breakfast Sandwiches: Egg & Cheese & Sausage, 1	66	4
Sandwiches: Bagel: Chicken Fajita, 1	74	
Sandwiches: Bagel: Smoked Salmon, 1	74	
Sandwiches: Bagel: Garden Veggie, 1	80	7
Sandwiches: Bagel: Herby Turkey, 1	73	4
Sandwiches: Bagel: Santa Fe Turkey, 1	71	4
Sandwiches: Deli: Chicken Breast, 1	62	4
Sandwiches: Deli: Chicken Salad w. mayo, 1	67	4
Sandwiches: Deli: Ham w. mustard, 1	77	4
Sandwiches: Deli: Turkey w. Mayonnaise, 1	65	4

Burger King®

	C	F
Croissan'wich® with Sausage, Egg & Cheese, 1 each	26	1
Croissan'wich® with Sausage & Cheese, 1 each	24	1
Biscuit, 1 each	35	<1
Biscuit with Egg, 1 each	37	<1
Biscuit with Sausage, 1 each	35	1
Biscuit with Sausage, Egg & Cheese, 1 each	38	1
French Toast Sticks, 5 sticks	46	2
Cini-minis without Icing, 4 rolls	51	1
Hash Brown Rounds, small	23	2
Hash Brown Rounds, large	38	4
Bacon, 3 pieces	0	0
Ham, 2 pieces	0	0
Sausage Patty, 2 oz	0	0
Biscuit, 1 each	35	0
Grape Jam, 1 serving	7	0
Strawberry Jam, 1 serving	7	0

	C	F
Breakfast Syrup, 1 serving	21	0
Land O' Lakes® Whipped Classic Blend, 1 serving	0	0
Vanilla Icing (for Cini-minis), 1 serving	20	0
Whopper®, 1 each	53	4
Whopper® without Mayo, 1 each	53	4
Whopper® with Cheese, 1 each	55	4
Whopper® w/ Cheese w/o Mayo, 1 each	54	4
Double Whopper®, 1 each	53	4
Double Whopper® w/o Mayo, 1 each	53	4
Double Whopper® w/ Cheese, 1 each	55	4
Double Whopper® w/ Cheese w/o Mayo, 1 each	54	4
Whopper® Jr., 1 each	32	2
Whopper® Jr. without Mayo, 1 each	32	2
Whopper® Jr. with Cheese, 1 each	33	2
Whopper® Patty, 1 each	0	0
Whopper® Bun, 1 each	46	3
Hamburger Patty, 1 each	0	0
Hamburger Bun, 1 each	28	2
BK Broiler® Chicken Breast Patty, 1 each	4	<1
Bull's-Eye™ BBQ Sauce, 0.5 oz	5	NA
Ketchup, 0.5 oz	4	0
Lettuce, 0.75 oz	0	0
Mustard, ⅛ oz	0	0
Onion, 0.5 oz	1	0
Pickles, 4 slices	0	0
Processed American Cheese, 2 slices	1	0
Tartar Sauce, 0.5 oz	0	0
Tomato, 2 slices	1	0
Barbecue Dipping Sauce, 1 serving	9	0
Honey Flavored Dipping Sauce, 1 serving	23	0
Honey Mustard Dipping Sauce, 1 serving	9	0
Marinara Dipping Sauce, 1 serving	5	0
Ranch Dipping Sauce, 1 serving	1	0

	C	F
Sweet and Sour Dipping Sauce, 1 serving	10	0
Vanilla Shake, small	61	1
Vanilla Shake, medium	79	2
Chocolate Shake, small	62	3
Chocolate Shake, syrup added, small	77	2
Chocolate Shake, medium	80	4
Chocolate Shake, syrup added, medium	95	3
Strawberry Shake, syrup added, small	76	1
Strawberry Shake, syrup added, medium	95	2
Frozen Coca Cola® Classic, medium	92	0
Frozen Coca Cola® Classic, large	116	0
Frozen Minute Maid® Cherry, medium	92	0
Frozen Minute Maid® Cherry, large	116	0
Tropicana® Pure Orange Juice, 1 serving	33	0
Dutch Apple Pie, 1 each	52	1
Hershey's® Sundae Pie, 1 each	33	<1
Bull's-Eye™ BBQ Deluxe w/ or w/o Mayo, 1 each	30	2
Bull's-Eye™ BBQ Deluxe, 1 each	30	2
Hamburger, 1 each	30	2
Cheeseburger, 1 each	31	2
Double Hamburger, 1 each	30	2
Double Cheeseburger, 1 each	32	2
Bacon Double Cheeseburger, 1 each	32	2
BK Veggie with mayo, 1 each	45	4
BK Big Fish® Sandwich, 1 each	67	4
BK Broiler® Chicken Sandwich, 1 each	52	3
BK Broiler® Chicken Sandwich w/o Mayo, 1 each	51	3
Chicken Sandwich, 1 each	53	3
Chicken Sandwich w/o Mayo, 1 each	52	3
Chicken Tenders® Sandwich, 1 each	37	2
Chicken Tenders® Sandwich w/o Mayo, 1 each	36	2

	C	F
Chicken Club Sandwich, 1 each	55	4
Chicken Club Sandwich w/o Mayo, 1 each	54	4
Chicken Tenders®, 4 pieces	10	0
Chicken Tenders®, 5 pieces	13	<1
Chicken Tenders®, 6 pieces	15	<1
Chicken Tenders®, 8 pieces	20	<1
French Fries, no salt, small	29	2
French Fries, no salt, medium	46	4
French Fries, no salt, large	63	5
French Fries, no salt, king size	76	6
Onion Rings, child's	46	4
Onion Rings, medium	40	3
Onion Rings, large	60	5
Onion Rings, king size	70	5
Jalapeño Poppers®, 4 pieces	22	2
Mozzarella Sticks, 4 pieces	25	<1

Burgerville®

	C
Hamburger, Regular, 1 serving	29
Cheeseburger, Regular, 1 serving	29
Cheeseburger: Double Beef, 1 serving	29
Hamburger, Half Pound Colossal, 1 serving	31
Hamburger, Colossal, 1 serving	30
Cheeseburger: Tillamook, 1 serving	32
Cheeseburger: Pepper Bacon, 1 serving	28
Gardenburger, Regular, 1 serving	53
Gardenburger: Spicy Black Bean, 1 serving	45
Turkey Burger, 1 serving	33
Turkey Club Sandwich, 1 serving	38
Chicken: Deluxe Crispy Chicken, 1 serving	56
Chicken: Crispy Chicken, 1 serving	55
Chicken: Grilled Chicken, 1 serving	45
Halibut Fillet Sandwich, 1 serving	42
Halibut Fish, 3 pieces, 1 serving	25
Chicken Strips, 5 pieces, 1 serving	36

	C	F
Protein Platter, 1 serving	6	
French Fries: 5 oz, regular	44	
French Fries: 6 oz, large	57	

Carl's Jr.®

	C	F
Southwest Spicy Chicken Sandwich, 1 each	48	2
Charbroiled Sirloin Steak Sandwich, 1 each	52	2
Carl's Catch Fish Sandwich, 1 each	55	2
American Cheese, large	1	0
Swiss-Style Cheese, 1 serving	0	0
French Fries, kids	32	2
French Fries, small	37	3
French Fries, medium	59	5
French Fries, large	80	6
Onion Rings, 1 serving	53	3
Zucchini, 1 serving	31	2
CrissCut Fries®, 1 serving	43	4
Chicken Stars, 6 pieces	14	<1
Potato Broccoli and Cheese, 1 serving	76	6
Potato Bacon and Cheese, 1 serving	75	6
Plain Potato without Margarine, 1 serving	68	6
Potato Sour Cream and Chives, 1 serving	70	6
Charbroiled Chicken Salad-to-Go, 1 serving	12	4
Garden Salad-to-Go™, 1 serving	4	2
House Dressing, 1 serving	3	0
Blue Cheese Dressing, 1 serving	1	0
1000 Island Dressing, 1 serving	5	0
Fat Free Italian Dressing, 1 serving	4	0
Fat Free French Dressing, 1 serving	16	<1
Croutons, 1 serving	5	0
Breadsticks, 1 serving	7	<1
Salsa, 1 serving	2	0
Mustard Sauce, 1 serving	11	0
Honey Sauce, 1 serving	22	0

	C	F
BBQ Sauce, 1 serving	11	0
Chocolate Chip Cookie, 1 serving	46	1
Chocolate Cake, 1 serving	48	1
Strawberry Swirl Cheesecake, 1 serving	30	0
Sourdough Breakfast, 1 serving	33	1
Sunrise Sandwich® (no meat), 1 serving	28	<1
Breakfast Burrito, 1 serving	36	1
French Toast Dips® (w/o syrup), 1 serving	42	1
Breakfast Quesadilla, 1 serving	38	1
Scrambled Eggs, 1 serving	1	0
English Muffin with Margarine, 1 serving	28	2
Bacon, 2 strips	0	0
Sausage, 1 patty	2	0
Hash Brown Nuggets, 1 serving	32	2
Blueberry Muffin, 1 each	49	1
Bran Raisin Muffin, 1 each	61	6
Cheese Danish, 1 serving	49	1
Table Syrup, 1 serving	21	0
Grape Jelly, 1 serving	9	0
Strawberry Jam, 1 serving	9	0
Carl's Famous Star®, 1 each	50	3
Super Star®, 1 each	51	3
Sourdough Bacon Cheeseburger, 1 each	37	2
Sourdough Ranch Bacon Cheeseburger, 1 each	43	3
Double Sourdough Bacon Cheeseburger, 1 each	37	2
Western Bacon Cheeseburger, 1 each	64	3
Double Western Bacon Cheeseburger®, 1 each	65	3
Famous Bacon Cheeseburger™, 1 each	51	3
Hamburger, 1 each	36	1
Charbroiled BBQ Chicken Sandwich, 1 each	41	2
Charbroiled BBQ Club Sandwich, 1 each	37	2

	C	F
Charbroiled Santa Fe Chicken Sandwich™, 1 each	37	2
Carl's Ranch Crispy Chicken Sandwich, 1 each	71	3
Carl's Bacon Swiss Crispy Chicken Sandwich, 1 each	72	3
Carl's Western Bacon Crispy Chicken Sandwich, 1 each	91	3
Spicy Chicken Sandwich, 1 each	47	2
Orange Juice, 1 serving	37	0
Milk (1% fat), 1 serving	18	0
Vanilla Shake, small	78	0
Chocolate Shake, small	96	0
Strawberry Shake, small	91	0
Vanilla Shake, regular	115	0
Chocolate Shake, regular	140	<1
Strawberry Shake, regular	133	0
Raspberry Nestea, regular	42	0
Iced Tea, 1 serving	0	0
Hot Chocolate, 1 serving	22	1

Caribou Coffee®

	C	F
Alaskan Fruit Smoothies: Creampop (2% milk), 16 fl oz	66	
Alaskan Fruit Smoothies: Passion Green Tea (2% milk), 16 fl oz	48	
Alaskan Fruit Smoothies: Strawberry Banana (2% milk), 16 fl oz	65	
Alaskan Fruit Smoothies: Wildberry (2% milk), 16 fl oz	57	
Coffee Coolers: Caramel (2% milk), 16 fl oz	87	
Coffee Coolers: Chocolate (2% milk), 16 fl oz	61	
Coffee Coolers: Espresso, Coffee (2% milk) average, 16 fl oz	47	
Coffee Coolers: Mint Oreo (2% milk), 16 fl oz	85	
Coffee Coolers: Vanilla (2% milk), 16 fl oz	63	
Espresso: Breve (2% milk), 16 fl oz	14	
Espresso: Campfire Mocha (2% milk), 16 fl oz	97	

	C	F
Espresso: Cappuccino (2% milk), 16 fl oz	18	
Espresso: Espresso (2% milk), 16 fl oz	2	
Espresso: Latte (2% milk), 16 fl oz	20	
Espresso: Macchiato (2% milk), 16 fl oz	2	
Espresso: Mocha (2% milk), 16 fl oz	63	
Espresso: White Chocolate Mocha (2% milk), 16 fl oz	39	
Skinny Bou Latte: Low Calorie (2% milk), 16 fl oz	17	
Skinny Bou Latte: Low Carb (2% milk), 16 fl oz	10	
Wild: Caramel Highrise (2% milk), 16 fl oz	55	
Wild: Hot Apple Blast (2% milk), 16 fl oz	84	
Wild: Lite White Berry (2% milk), 16 fl oz	94	
Wild: Mint Condition (2% milk), 16 fl oz	89	

Chevys Fresh Mex®

	C	F
Burritos: All Veggies and Pico de Gallo w/ Ranchero Sauce, 1	49	
Catch of the Day: Fresh Fish, San Antonio Veges, Salsa & Tomalito, 1	16	
Fajitas: Chicken w/ San Antonio Veges & Tomalito, 1	13	
Fajitas: Shrimp w/ San Antonio Veges & Tomalito, 1	13	
Fajitas: Marinated Veges w/ San Antonio Veges & Tomalito, 1	16	
Salad: Grilled Chicken w/ Salsa Vinaigrette Dressing, 1	53	
Salad: Mixed Green, 1	42	
Sides: Black Beans, 1	11	
Sides: Guacamole, 2 oz	3	
Sides: Mexican Rice, 1	39	
Sides: Salsa for Chips, 5 oz	8	
Sides: Sour Cream, 1	2	

	C	F
Sides: Tortilla, Corn, 1	17	
Sides: Tortilla, El Machino, 1	27	

Chi-Chi's ®

APPETIZERS

	C	F
Beef and Bean Nachos without Guacamole, 1 order	78	15
Buffalo Chicken Strips, 1 order	38	2.3
Cheese Nachos without Guacamole, 1 order	49	6.8
Chicken Nachos without Guacmole, 1 order	55	6.9
Chile Con Queso, 1 order	75	4.4
Fiesta Platter, 1 order	155	6.7
Mexican Springrolls, 1 order	77	6.7
Pepper Jack Cheese Wedges, 1 order	62	1
Seafood Nachos without Guacamole, 1 order	69	5
Texas Nachos, 1 order	164	19.5
Tex-Mex BBQ Wings, 1 order	51	5

BURRITOS

	C	F
El Grande Burrito, Beef, 1 order	133	15
El Grande Burrito, Chicken, 1 order	133	13.6
El Grande Burrito, Seafood, 1 order	149	13
El Grande Burrito, Suprema, 1 order	146	15.4
Outrageous Burrito, 1 order	309	27.2
Twice Grilled BBQ Burrito, Chicken, 1 order	174	16.8
Twice Grilled BBQ Burrito, Steak, 1 order	168	16.8

CHIMICHANGAS

	C	F
Beef, 1 order	139	16.1
Chicken, 1 order	138	15.2
Seafood, 1 order	154	14.6
Suprema, 1 order	144	14.8

ENCHILADAS

	C	F
Chicken Enchiladas Suprema, 1 order	133	12.6
Enchiladas Cancun, 1 order	149	12.5
Enchiladas Conquistador, Beef, 1 order	87	11.9

	C	F
Enchiladas Conquistador, Chicken, 1 order	88	11.1
Enchiladas Tampico, 1 order	89	12.2
Lobster Enchiladas, 1 order	137	20.1
Tres Amigos Enchiladas, 1 order	90	12.1

FAJITAS

	C	F
Blackened Chicken Fajitas, 1 order	176	21
Grilled Chicken Fajitas, 1 order	168	18.4
Grilled Shrimp Fajitas, 1 order	161	18.4
Grilled Skirt Steak Fajitas, 1 order	162	18.4
Seared Vegetable Fajitas, 1 order	171	22.3
Steak and Chicken Fajitas, 1 order	165	18.4

QUESADILLAS

	C	F
Blackened Chicken Quesadilla, 1 order	75	6.3
Cheese Quesadilla, 1 order	65	5
Grilled Chicken Quesadilla, 1 order	67	4
Steak and Mushroom Quesadilla, 1 order	87	6

MAIN ENTREES

	C	F
Acapulco Chicken, 1 order	74	6.5
Buffalo Chicken Sandwich, 1 order	107	6.3
Chicken Sandwich, 1 order	94	6.3
Elegante Combo, 1 order	144	17.4
Ground Chuck Burger, 1 order	85	6.3
Hacienda Steak, 1 order	80	6.2
Mazatlan Seafood Platter, 1 order	186	16.8
Mucho Carne Dinner, 1 order	153	19.5
Pollo Magnifico, 1 order	97	5.9
Shrimp Diablo, 1 order	62	4.1
Tamales Rancheros, 1 order	180	21.3

MISCELLANEOUS

	C	F
Chili-Cheddar Mashed Potatoes, 1 order	24	2
Hot Garden Salsa, 1 order	9	1.2
Mexican Rice, 1 order	34	1
Original Mild Salsa, 1 order	3	1
Refried Beans, 1 order	28	8.7
San Antonio Chili, 1 order	32	7.2

	C	F
Southwestern Veggie Medley, Sauteed, 1 order	9	2.3
Southwestern Veggie Medley, Steamed, 1 order	7	2.2
Sweet Corn Cake, 1 order	15	0.6
Tortilla Soup, 1 order	58	11.2

KIDS

	C	F
Amigo Burger, 1 order	65	2
Cheese Pizza, 1 order	80	4
Chi-Chi's Dog, 1 order	61	4
Chicken Strips, 1 order	56	2
Corndog, 1 order	35	3
Fiesta Sundae, 1 order	62	0
Macaroni & Cheese, 1 order	82	4
Nino Burrito, Bean, 1 order	53	6.2
Nino Burrito, Beef, 1 order	43	4
Nino Burrito, Chicken, 1 order	45	2.5
Senor Taco, Beef, 1 order	54	5
Senor Taco, Chicken, 1 order	56	4.6

LOW FAT

	C	F
Acapulco Chicken, 1 order	42	7.6
Chicken Enchiladas, 1 order	98	8
Chicken Soft Tacos, 1 order	88	7
Chicken Tortilla Soup, 1 order	47	9.8
Santa Fe Grilled Chicken Salad, 1 order	25	6.5

DESSERTS

	C	F
Mexican Fried Ice Cream with Caramel, 1 order	120	2.7
Mexican Fried Ice Cream with Chocolate Syrup, 1 order	116	2.7
Mexican Fried Ice Cream with Honey, 1 order	122	2.7
Mexican Fried Ice Cream with Strawberry Syrup, 1 order	107	3.1
Molten Meltdown Cake, 1 piece	78	2

Chick-Fil-A®

	C	F
Sandwich: Chicken Sandwich, 1 sandwich	38	

	C	F
Sandwich: Chargrilled Chicken Sandwich, 1 sandwich	33	
Sandwich: Chicken Salad Sandwich, 1 sandwich	32	
Cool Wraps®: Chicken Caesar, 1 wrap	52	
Cool Wraps®: Chargrilled/Spicy Chicken, average, 1 wrap	54	
Breakfast: Plain Biscuit, 1 biscuit	38	
Breakfast: Biscuit and Gravy, 1 biscuit	44	
Breakfast: Biscuit: w. Bacon, Egg & Cheese, 1 biscuit	39	
Breakfast: Biscuit: w. Sausage, Egg & Cheese, 1 biscuit	45	
Breakfast: Hashbrowns, 1 serving	25	
Breakfast: Chiick-n-Minis, 3 count, 1 serving	28	
Breakfast: Chicken Biscuit, 1 serving	44	
Breakfast: Chicken Platter, 1 serving	51	
Breakfast: Bacon Platter, 1 serving	44	
Breakfast: Chicken Burrito, 1 serving	39	
Breakfast: Sausage Burrito, 1 serving	40	
Breakfast: Chicken, Egg & Cheese Bagel, 1 serving	47	
Salads: Chick-n-Strips®, 1 serving	22	
Salads: Chargrilled Chicken Garden, 1 serving	9	
Salads: Southwest Chargrilled Chicken, 1 serving	17	
Salad Dressing: Caesar Dressing, 1 serving	1	
Salad Dressing: Bleu Cheese; Buttermilk, 1 serving	15	
Salad Dressing: Fat Free Honey Mustard, 1 serving	1	
Salad Dressing: Light Italian Dressing, 1 serving	14	
Salad Dressing: Spicy Dressing, 1 serving	22	
Salad Dressing: Thousand Island, 1 serving	5	
Chicken, Nuggets: (8-pack), 1 serving	12	
Chicken, Chick-n-Strips* (4-count), 1 serving	14	

	C	F
Dipping Sauces: Polynesian, 1 oz	13	
Dipping Sauces: Barbecue; Honey Mustard, average, 1 oz	10	
Dipping Sauces: Buffalo Sauce ¾ oz	1	
Sides: Carrot & Raisin Salad, small	28	
Sides: Fresh Fruit Cups, 4 oz	16	
Sides: Coleslaw, small, 1 serving	17	
Sides: Garlic and Butter Croutons, 1 serving	64	
Sides: Side Salad, 1 serving	9	
Sides: Tortilla Strips, 1 serving	44	
Sides: Waffle Potato Fries, 1 serving	30	
Desserts: Cheesecake, 3.3 oz slice, 1 serving	38	
Desserts: Icedream® Cone, small, 1 serving	28	
Desserts: Lemon Pie, 4 oz slice, 1 serving	51	
Desserts: Fudge Nut Brownie (1), 1 serving	45	

Chili's®

	C	F
Starters: Awesome Blossom w. Sauce, 1	191	
Starters: Vt Whole w. Blossom Sauce, 1	48	
Starters: Boneless Buffalo Wings + Sauce, 1	64	
Starters: Boneless Shanghai Wings, 1	90	
Starters: Fajita Nachos: Chicken, 1	94	
Starters: Fajita Nachos: Beef, 1	100	
Starters: Buffalo Wings w. Dressing, 1	5	
Guiltless Grill: Chicken Platter, 1	83	
Guiltless Grill: Chicken Grill Pita, 1	77	
Guiltless Grill: Chicken Sandwich, 1	70	
Guiltless Grill: Tomato Basil Pasta, 1	106	
Burgers: Ranch (no fries), 1	64	
Burgers: Chipotle Bleu Chse Bacon (no fries), 1	54	
Burgers: Grnd Peppercorn w. Strings, Dr (no fries), 1	78	
Burgers: Bunless: Old Timer, 1	11	

	C	F
Burgers: Bunless: Mushroom Swiss w. Mayo, 1	14	
Meals: Chili's Filet, 1	69	
Meals: Bottomless Tostada Chips w. Salsa, 1	109	
Meals: Cajun Chicken Pasta, 1	103	
Meals: Cajun Chicken Sandwich, 1	77	
Meals: Cheese Steak Sandwich (no fries), 1	67	
Meals: Chicken Caesar Pita (no fries), 1	33	
Meals: Citrus Fire Chicken & Shrimp, 1	73	
Meals: Country Fried Steak, 1	126	
Meals: Flame Grilled Rib Eye, 1	70	
Meals: Ginger Citrus Glazed Salmon, 1	70	
Meals: Grilled Baby Back Ribs, 1	109	
Meals: Grilled Shrimp Alfredo, 1	142	
Meals: Hawaiian Steak, 1	88	
Meals: Margarita Grilled Chicken, 1	72	
Meals: Margarita Grilled Tuna, 1	97	
Meals: South Western Egg Rolls, 1	86	
Meals: Veggie & Smoked Chse Quesadilla, 1	95	
Fajitas: Mushroom Jack (3 Tortillas & Garnishes), 1	103	
Fajitas: Chicken (3 Tortillas & Garnishes), 1	97	
Fajitas: Steak (3 Tortillas & Garnishes), 1	93	
Fajitas: Knife & Fork Beef & Chkn Combo, no tortilla (w. veggies, sour cream, pica de gallo, guacamole), 1	17	
Fajitas: Knife & Fork Chicken Fajitas, no tortilla (w. veggies, sour cream, pica de gallo, guacamole), 1	17	
Salad: Chicken Fajita Caesar w/ dressing, 1	11	
Salad: Dinner Caesar w/ dressing, 1	5	
Salad: Dinner House Salad w. Ranch dressing, 1	8	
Salad: Quesadilla Explosion w/dressing, 1	68	

	C	F
Desserts: Choc Chip Paradise Pie, 1 slice	188	
Desserts: Molten Choc Cake, 1 slice	207	

Chipotle®

	C	F
Tortillas, 13" Flour, 1	55	5
Tortillas, 6" Flour, 3	48	6
Taco Shells, Crispy, 4	34	2
Rice, 5 oz	40	0
Beans, Black, 4 oz	22	0
Beans, Pinto, 4 oz	23	0
Fajita Vegetables, 3 oz	6	1
Barbacoa, 5 oz	1	0
Carnitas, 4 oz	0	0
Chicken, 4 oz	0	0
Steak, 4 oz	2	0
Salsa, Tomato, 4 oz	6	1
Salsa, Corn, 4 oz	22	3
Tomatillo, Red, 2 oz	4	0
Tomatillo, Green, 2 oz	3	0
Cheese, 1 oz	0	0
Sour Cream, 2 oz	2	0
Guacamole, 4 oz	8	5
Lettuce, 1 oz	0	0
Chips, 4 oz	71	5
Vinaigrette, 1 oz	11	0

Chuck E. Cheese®

	C	F
Appetizer, Buffalo Wings, 1 order	3	
Appetizer, French Fries, 1 order	37	
Appetizer, French Fries ala Carte, 1 order	37	
Appetizer, Italian Bread Sticks, 1 stick	27	
Appetizer, Sargento Mozzarella Sticks, 1 stick	7	
Pizza: medium, 1 slice	43	
Pizza: medium, BBQ Chicken, 1 slice	33	
Pizza: medium, Cheese, 1 slice	33	

	C	F
Pizza: medium, Pepperoni, 1 slice	36	
Pizza: medium, Vegetarian, 1 slice	70	
Sandwiches: Ham S Cheese, 1 sandwich	70	
Sandwiches: Grilled Chicken Sub, 1 sandwich	69	
Sandwiches: Italian Sub, 1 sandwich	27	
Sandwiches: Hot Dog, 1 sandwich	28	
Sandwiches: Hot Dog w. Cheese, 1 sandwich	45	
Birthday Cakes: 8" Chocolate White, ⅒ 8" cake	44	

Church's Chicken®

	C	F
Fried Chicken, Breast w. Skin, 1 piece	4	
Fried Chicken, Leg w. Skin, 1 piece	2	
Fried Chicken, Thigh w. Skin, 1 piece	5	
Fried Chicken, Crunchy Tenders, 1 piece	11	
Fried Chicken, Wing w. Skin, 1 piece	8	
Fried Chicken, Tender Crunchers, 6–8 pieces	32	
Side Items: Apple Pie, 3 oz	41	
Side Items: Honey Butter Biscuits, 1 biscuit	26	
Side Items: Cajun Rice, regular, 3 oz, 1 serving	16	
Side Items: Chicken Fried Steak w. Gravy, 1 serving	36	
Side Items: Cole Slaw, regular, 3 oz, 1 serving	8	
Side Items: Corn on the Cob, 1 ear, 1 serving	24	
Side Items: French Fries, regular, 1 serving	29	
Side Items: Mashed Potatoes & Gravy, reg., 1 serving	14	

Cinnabon®

	C	F
Classic, 1 roll	117	
Caramel Pecanbon, 1 roll, 1 roll	141	
Minibon, 1 roll, 1 roll	49	

	C	F
MiniBon, Strawberry, 1 roll	45	
CinnaPretzel, 1 pretzel	156	
CinnaPoppers (3), 1 order	41	
Cinnabon Stix (5), 1 order	54	
Drinks, Frusia, 12 fl. oz	38	
Drinks, Mochalata Chill, 12 fl. oz	62	

Cold Stone Creamery®

	C	F
Sweet Cream Ice Cream, Like It, average, all flavors, 1 serving	40	
Sweet Cream Ice Cream, Love It, average, all flavors, 1 serving	67	
Sweet Cream Ice Cream, Gotta Have It, average, all flavors, 1 serving	93	
Sweet Cream Ice Cream, Cake Batter, Like It, 1 serving	48	
Sweet Cream Ice Cream, Oreo Cookie, Like It, 1 serving	46	
Low Fat Frozen Yogurt, Chocolate, Like It, 1 serving	48	
Low Fat Frozen Yogurt, Chocolate, Love It, 1 serving	79	
Non Fat Frozen Yogurt: Like It, 1 serving	48	
Non Fat Frozen Yogurt: Love It, average all flavors, 1 serving	80	
Non Fat Frozen Yogurt: Gotta Have It, average all flavors, 1 serving	113	
Sinless Sorbet, Like It, 1 serving	50	
Sinless Sorbet, Love It, 1 serving	84	
Sinless Sorbet, Gotta Have It, 1 serving	118	
Ice Cream Cake, ⅛ small round cake, Butterfinger Bonanza, 1 slice	58	
Ice Cream Cake, ⅛ small round cake, Celebration Sensation, 1 slice	46	
Ice Cream Cake, ⅛ small round cake, Cheesecake Named Desire, 1 slice	57	
Ice Cream Cake, ⅛ small round cake, Chocolate Chipper, 1 slice	50	

	C	F
Ice Cream Cake, ⅛ small round cake, Midnight Delight, 1 slice	61	
Ice Cream Cake, ⅛ small round cake, Peanut Butter, 1 slice	54	
Ice Cream Cake, ⅛ small round cake, Strawberry Passion, 1 slice	50	
Ice Cream Cake, ⅛ small round cake, Zebra Stripes Dark, 1 slice	54	
Waffle cone or bowl, 1 serving	29	

Corner Bakery Cafe ®

BREAKFAST

	C	F
All American Scrambler, 1 order	2	0
Baked French Toast, 1 order	146	8
Farmer's Scrambler, 1 order	2	0
Fruit Medley, 1 order	26	3
Mixed Berry Parfait, 1 order	68	10
Oatmeal, 1 order	39	6
Sunrise Scrambler, 1 order	2	0
Swiss Oatmeal, 1 order	73	12
The Commuter Croissant, 1 order	60	4

PANINI

	C	F
Chicken Pomodori Panini, 1 sandwich	92	6
Club Panini, 1 sandwich	79	4
Corned Beef Reuben Panini, 1 sandwich	105	11
Grilled Ham and Swiss Panini, 1 sandwich	91	7
Ham and Cheddar Panini, 1 sandwich	48	4
Smoked Bacon and Cheddar Panini, 1 sandwich	57	4

PASTA

	C	F
Chicken Carbonara pasta, 1 order	94	7
Penne pasta with Marinara, 1 order	106	9
Pesto Cavatappi pasta, 1 order	96	9
Half Moon Cheese Ravioli, 1 order	73	7

SALADS & DRESSINGS

	C	F
Caesar salad dressing, 2 oz	2	0
Ranch salad dressing, 2 oz	2	0

	C	F
Balsamic Vinaigrette salad dressing, 2 oz	4	0
Caesar Entree Salad, 1 order	51	8
Caesar Entree Salad w/ Roasted Chicken (no croutons), 1 order	14	5
Caesar Entree Salad w/ Roasted Chicken and Croutons, 1 order	39	5
Cavatappi Pasta Salad, 1 order	35	4
Chopped Entree Salad, 1 order	7	2
D.C. Chicken Salad, 1 order	20	8
Egg Salad, 1 order	2	1
Golden Pineapple Salad, 1 order	19	2
Harvest Entree Salad, 1 order	43	13
Harvest Entree Salad with Roasted Chicken, 1 order	81	20
Potato Dill Salad, 1 order	24	5
Sante Fe Ranch Entree Salad, 1 order	41	9
Tuna Salad, 1 order	3	2

SANDWICHES

	C	F
Chicken Pesto Sandwich, 1 sandwich	105	6
Ham on Pretzel Sandwich, 1 sandwich	50	6
Southwest Roast Beef Sandwich, 1 sandwich	61	11
Tomato Mozzarella Sandwich, 1 sandwich	86	8
Tuna Salad Sandwich on Olive Bread, 1 sandwich	78	9
Turkey Derby Sandwich, 1 sandwich	74	11
Turkey Swiss Sandwich (No Mayo), 1 sandwich	72	10
Uptown Turkey Sandwich, 1 sandwich	71	11

SOUPS

	C	F
Big Al's Chili, 15 oz (bowl), 1 serving	35	10
Big Al's Chili, 10 oz (cup), 1 serving	23	7
Cheddar Broccoli Soup, 15 oz (bowl), 1 serving	25	2.5
Cheddar Broccoli Soup, 10 oz (cup), 1 serving	17	1.5
Loaded Baked Potato Soup, 15 oz (bowl), 1 serving	40	3

	C	F
Loaded Baked Potato Soup, 10 oz (cup), 1 serving	27	2
Mom's Chicken Noodle Soup, 15 oz (bowl), 1 serving	30	2.5
Mom's Chicken Noodle Soup, 10 oz (cup), 1 serving	20	1.5
Roasted Tomato Basil Soup, 15 oz (bowl), 1 serving	38	5
Roasted Tomato Basil Soup, 10 oz (cup), 1 serving	25	3
Southwest Corn Chowder, 15 oz (bowl), 1 serving	45	3
Southwest Corn Chowder, 10 oz (cup), 1 serving	30	2
Zesty Chicken Tortilla Soup, 15 oz (bowl), 1 serving	32	7.5
Zesty Chicken Tortilla Soup, 10 oz (cup), 1 serving	22	5

Dairy Queen®

	C	F
Peanut Buster Parfait, 1 serving	99	2
Pecan Mudslide® Treat, 1 serving	85	2
Strawberry Shortcake, 1 serving	70	1
Brownie Earthquake®, 1 serving	112	0
DQ® Sandwich, 1 serving	31	1
Chocolate Dilly® Bar, 1 serving	21	0
Buster Bar®, 1 serving	41	2
Starkiss®, 1 serving	21	0
DQ® Fudge Bar, no sugar added, 1 serving	13	0
DQ® Vanilla Orange Bar, no sugar add., 1 serving	17	0
Lemon DQ® Freez'r, 0.5 cup	20	0
Blizzard® Chocolate Sandwich Cookie, small	79	1
Blizzard® Chocolate Chip Cookie, medium	97	1
Blizzard® Dough, small	99	1
Blizzard® Chocolate Chip Cookie, medium	143	2
Heath® DQ Treatzza Pizza®, ⅛ of pizza	28	1
M&M's® DQ Treatzza Pizza®, ⅛ of pizza	29	1

	C	F
DQ® Frozen 8" Round Cake, ⅛ of cake	56	<1
DQ® Layered 8" Round Cake, ⅛ of cake	49	0
DQ Homestyle® Hamburger, 1 each	29	2
DQ Homestyle® Cheeseburger, 1 each	29	2
DQ Homestyle® Double Cheeseburger, 1 each	30	2
DQ Homestyle® Bacon Double Cheeseburger, 1 each	31	2
DQ Ultimate® Burger, 1 each	29	2
Hot Dog, 1 each	19	1
Chili 'n' Cheese Dog, 1 each	22	2
Chicken Breast Fillet Sandwich, 1 each	48	4
Grilled Chicken Sandwich, 1 each	30	3
Chicken Strip Basket™, 1 each	102	5
DQ® Vanilla Soft Serve, 0.5 cup	22	0
DQ® Chocolate Soft Serve, 0.5 cup	22	0
Vanilla Cone, small	38	0
Vanilla Cone, medium	53	0
Vanilla Cone, large	65	0
Chocolate Cone, small	37	0
Chocolate Cone, medium	53	0
Dipped Cone, small	42	1
Dipped Cone, medium	59	1
Chocolate Malt, small	111	0
Chocolate Malt, medium	153	0
Chocolate Shake, small	94	0
Chocolate Shake, medium	130	0
Frozen Hot Chocolate, 1 serving	127	3
Misty® Slush, small	56	0
Misty® Slush, medium	74	0
Chocolate Sundae, small	49	0
Chocolate Sundae, medium	71	0
Banana Split, 1 serving	96	3
Crispy Chicken Salad with Honey Mustard Dressing, 1 each	36	6
Crispy Chicken Salad with Fat Free Italian Dressing, 1 each	27	6

	C	F
Grilled Chicken Salad with Honey Mustard Dressing, 1 each	22	3
Grilled Chicken Salad with Fat Free Italian Dressing, 1 each	13	3
French Fries, small	42	3
French Fries, medium	53	4
Onion Rings, 1 serving	39	3

Denny's®

	C
Breakfast, Corned Beef Hash Slam, no bread, 1 serving	11
Breakfast, Pancakes (3), no syrup/ marg., 2 pancakes	47
Breakfast, Country Scramble, no syrup/marg., 1 serving	79
Breakfast, Two Egg Breakfast w. hash browns, 1 serving	20
Breakfast, All American Slam, no toast, 1 serving	3
Breakfast, French Slam, no syrup/ marg., 1 serving	74
Breakfast, Grand Slam Slugger, no bread/potato, 1 serving	74
Breakfast, Lumberjack Slam, w. hash browns, 1 serving	73
Breakfast, Moons Over My Hammy, 1 serving	42
Breakfast, Original Grand Slam, no toast, 1 serving	33
Breakfast, Original Grand Slam, w/ syrup & Margarine, 1 serving	101
Soup, Chicken Noodle, 8 fl. oz	14
Soup, Vegetable Beef, 8 fl. oz	11
Sandwiches, Albacore Tuna Melt, (no fries/sauces), 1 sandwich	42
Sandwiches, BBQ Chicken, (no fries/ sauces), 1 sandwich	86
Sandwiches, BLT, (no fries/sauces), 1 sandwich	50
Sandwiches, Bacon Cheddar Burger, (no fries/sauces), 1 sandwich	58
Sandwiches, Boca Burger, (no fries/ sauces), 1 sandwich	64

	C	F
Sandwiches, Buffalo Chicken Sandwich, (no fries/sauces), 1 sandwich	80	
Sandwiches, Chicken Ranch Melt, (no fries/sauces), 1 sandwich	57	
Sandwiches, Classic Burger, (no fries/sauces), 1 sandwich	56	
Sandwiches, Club Sandwich, (no fries/sauces), 1 sandwich	45	
Sandwiches, Grilled Chicken, no Dressing, fries or sauce, 1 sandwich	56	
Sandwiches, Hoagie Chicken Melt, (no fries/sauces), 1 sandwich	43	
Sandwiches, HoagiePhillyMelt, (no fries/sauces), 1 sandwich	58	
Sandwiches, Mushroom Swiss Burger, (no fries/sauces), 1 sandwich	63	
Sandwiches, The Super Bird Sandwich, (no fries/sauces), 1 sandwich	32	
Sandwiches, Grilled Tilapia Dinner, (no fries/sauces), 1 sandwich	31	
Appetizers: No sides/condiments, Buffalo Wings (9), 9 wings	11	
Appetizers: No sides/condiments, Buffalo Chicken Strips (5), 5 strips	43	
Appetizers: No sides/condiments, Chicken Strips (5), 5 strips	56	
Entrees: No sides/condiments, Country Fried Steak, 1 serving	30	
Entrees: No sides/condiments, Fish & Chips, 1 serving	83	
Entrees: No sides/condiments, Fried Shrimp Dinner, 1 serving	18	
Entrees: No sides/condiments, Fried Shrimp & Shrimp Scampi, 1 serving	15	
Entrees: Grilled Chicken Dinner, 1 serving	15	
Entrees: No sides/condiments, Grilled Tilapia Dinner, 1 serving	31	
Appetizers: No sides/condiments, Mozzarella Sticks (8), 8 sticks	49	
Entrees: No sides/condiments, Roast Turkey & Stuffing w. Gravy, 1 serving	62	

	C	F
Appetizers: Sampler, no condiments, 1 serving	124	
Entrees: No sides/condiments, Shrimp Scampi Skillet Dinner, 1 serving	3	
Entrees: No sides/condiments, Sirloin Steak Dinner, 1 serving	1	
Appetizers: No sides/condiments, Smothered Cheese Fries, 1 serving	69	
Entrees: No sides/condiments, Steak & Shrimp Dinner, 1 serving	31	
Entrees: No sides/condiments, T-Bone Steak Dinner, 1 serving	0	
Sides, Garlic Bread, 2 pieces	5	
Sides, Corn in Butter Sauce, 3 oz	23	
Sides, Onion Rings, 4 oz	38	
Sides, Fries, unsalted, 6 oz	57	
Sides, Fries, seasoned, 4 oz	35	
Sides, Gravy, all types, average, 1 serving	2	
Sides, Green Beans in sauce, 3 oz	8	
Sides, Potato, baked, plain w/skin, 1 serving	51	
Sides, Potatoes, Mashed, 5 oz	23	
Salads, w/o dressing or bread, 1 serving	23	
Salads, w/o dressing or bread, Albacore Tuna, 1 serving	22	
Salads, w/o dressing or bread, Fried Chicken Strips, 1 serving	26	
Salads, Grilled Chicken Caesar w/ dressing, 1 serving	20	
Salads, w/o dressing or bread, Grilled Chicken Breast, 1 serving	10	
Salads, Side Caesar w/ dressing, 1 serving	20	
Salads, w/o dressing or bread, Side Garden, 1 serving	16	
Dressings & Sauces, BBQ, 1.5 oz	11	
Dressings & Sauces, Blue Cheese, 1 oz	1	
Dressings & Sauces, Caesar, Ranch, 1 oz	1	
Dressings & Sauces, French, regular, 1 oz	3	

	C	F
Dressings & Sauces, Honey Mustard, 1 oz	20	
Dressings & Sauces, Italian (low calorie), Salsa, 1 oz	3	
Dressings & Sauces, Marinara, 1.5 oz	7	
Dressings & Sauces, Sour Cream, 1.5 oz	2	
Dressings & Sauces, Tartar, 1.5 oz	3	
Dressings & Sauces, Thousand Island, 1 oz	5	
Desserts, Carrot Cake, 8 oz	99	
Desserts, Fudge Brownie, 10 oz	49	
Desserts, Apple Pie, ⅛ of whole pie, 7 oz	64	
Desserts, Cheesecake, no topping, 4 oz	51	
Desserts, Chocolate Peanut Butter, 6 oz	64	
Desserts, Sundaes, Banana Split, 1 serving	121	
Desserts, Sundaes, Single Scoop, no topping, 1 serving	14	
Desserts, Sundaes, Double Scoop, no topping, 1 serving	29	
Dessert Toppings, Chocolate, 2 oz	34	
Dessert Toppings, Blueberry, 3 oz	26	
Dessert Toppings, Fudge, 2 oz	30	
Dessert Toppings, Strawberry, 3 oz	26	
Drinks, Cappuccino, 8 fl oz	28	
Drinks, Floats, Root beer or Cola, 12 fl oz	47	
Drinks, Milkshake, Vanilla or Chocolate, 12 fl oz	76	
Drinks, Ruby Red Grapefruit Juice, 10 fl oz	41	
Drinks, Raspberry Iced Tea, 16 fl oz	21	

Domino's Pizza®

	C	F
Ultimate Deep Dish Pepperoni Pizza, 6 inch, 1 pizza	69	4
Ultimate Deep Dish Pepperoni Pizza, 12 inch (medium), quarter of pizza	56	3

	C	F
Ultimate Deep Dish Pepperoni Pizza, 14 inch (large), Quarter of pizza	81	5
Domino's Breadsticks, 1 piece	18	1
Domino's Buffalo Wings, Barbeque, 1 average piece	2	<1
Domino's Buffalo Wings, Hot Wings, 1 average piece	0.5	<1
Double Cheesy Bread, 1 piece	18	1
Classic Hand Tossed Cheese Pizza, 12 inch (medium), quarter of pizza	55	3
Classic Hand Tossed Cheese Pizza, 14 inch (large), quarter of pizza	75	4
Classic Hand Tossed Pepperoni Pizza, 12 inch (medium), quarter of pizza	55	3
Classic Hand Tossed Pepperoni Pizza, 14 inch (large), quarter of pizza	75	4
Crunchy Thin Crust Cheese Pizza, 12 inch (medium), quarter of pizza	31	2
Crunchy Thin Crust Cheese Pizza, 14 inch (large), quarter of pizza	43	2
Crunchy Thin Crust Pepperoni Pizza, 12 inch (medium), quarter of pizza	31	2
Crunchy Thin Crust Pepperoni Pizza, 14 inch (large), quarter of pizza	44	2
Ultimate Deep Dish Cheese Pizza, 12 inch (medium), quarter of pizza	68	4
Ultimate Deep Dish Cheese Pizza, 14 inch (large), quarter of pizza	56	3
Ultimate Deep Dish Cheese Pizza, 6 inch, quarter of pizza	80	5

Don Pablos®

	C	F
Appetizers, Beef Taquito, no garnish, 1 serving	5	
Appetizers, Buffalo Chicken Wings, 8 wings	43	
Appetizers, Chicken Flauta, no garnish, 1 serving	6	
Appetizers, Nachos, Taco Beef, 1 serving	85	
Appetizers, Nachos, Beef Fajita, 1 serving	71	
Appetizers, Nachos, Chicken Fajita, 1 serving	73	

	C	F
Quesadillas, incl. s. cream & guacamole, Cheese, 1 serving	105	
Quesadillas, incl. s. cream & guacamole, Mesquite Grilled Chicken, 1 serving	110	
Quesadillas, incl. s. cream & guacamole, Mesquite Grilled Steak, 1 serving	122	
Quesadillas, incl. s. cream & guacamole, Portabella Mush. & Veggie, 1 serving	136	
Quesadillas, incl. s. cream & guacamole, Primo Club, 1 serving	114	
Dips, no chips, Quesa Blanco, 1 cup	13	
Dips, no chips, Prairie Fire Bean w/cheese, 1 cup	23	
Dips, no chips, Spinach, 1 cup	8	
Burritos, w/o sides, 1 serving	70	
Burritos, w/o sides, 1 serving	123	
Chimichangas, w/rice & refritos, 1 serving	109	
Chimichangas, w/rice & refritos, 1 serving	71	
Rellenos, Beef, 1 serving	20	
Rellenos, Cheese, 1 serving	19	
Rellenos, Chicken, 1 serving	21	
Salads, Steak Fajita, 1 serving	27	
Salads, Chicken Fajita, 1 serving	28	
Salads, Traditional Taco, average, 1 serving	94	
Salad Dressing, Blue Cheese, 3 oz	3	
Salad Dressing, House Vinaigrette, 3 oz	10	
Salad Dressing, Honey Mustard, 3 oz	17	
Salad Dressing, Low Fat French, 3 oz	30	
Salad Dressing, Ranch, 3 oz	3	
Sides, Chips & Salsa, 1 serving	43	
Sides, Guacamole	2	
Sides, Mexican Rice, 3 oz	21	
Sides, Refritos, 5 oz	23	
Sides, Salsa, 1 oz	1	
Sides, Side Salad, 1 serving	8	
Sides, Sour Cream, 1.25 oz	2	

	C	F
Sides, Sour Cream, 1 oz	1	
Sides, Flour Tortilla, 7"	20	

Dunkin' Donuts®

	C	F
Bagel, Berry Berry, 1 bagel	69	4
Bagel, Blueberry, 1 bagel	69	2
Bagel, Cinnamon Raisin, 1 bagel	69	3
Bagel, Everything, 1 bagel	67	2
Bagel, Garlic, 1 bagel	68	2
Bagel, Onion, 1 bagel	66	3
Bagel, Plain, 1 bagel	67	2
Bagel, Poppyseed, 1 bagel	68	2
Bagel, Salt, 1 bagel	67	2
Bagel, Sesame, 1 bagel	74	0
Bagel, Sundried Tomato, 1 bagel	66	3
Bagel, Wheat, 1 bagel	67	4
Apple Cinnamon Pecan Muffin, 1 muffin	74	1
Banana Nut Muffin, 1 muffin	72	2
Blueberry Muffin, 1 muffin	76	2
Blueberry, Reduced Fat Muffin, 1 muffin	77	2
Chocolate Chip Muffin, 1 muffin	88	3
Coffee Cake Muffin, 1 muffin	102	2
Corn Muffin, 1 muffin	78	1
Cranberry Orange Muffin, 1 muffin	76	2
Honey Bran Raisin Muffin, 1 muffin	84	5
Lemon Poppyseed Muffin, 1 muffin	94	2
Éclair Donut, 1 each	39	<1
Glazed Cake, 1 each	33	<1
Glazed Chocolate Cruller, 1 each	35	1
Apple Fritter, 1 each	41	1
Biscuit, 1 each	32	<1
Coffee Roll, 1 each	33	1
Chocolate Frosted Coffee Roll, 1 each	36	1
Cinnamon Bun, 1 each	85	0
Croissant, Plain, 1 each	26	<1
Biscuit/Egg/Cheese Sandwich, 1 each	30	<1

	C	F
Biscuit/Sausage/Egg/Cheese Sandwich, 1 each	31	<1
English Muffin/Ham/Egg/Cheese, 1 each	31	2
Chocolate Chunk Cookie, 1 each	28	1
Chocolate Chunk with Nuts Cookie, 1 each	27	1
Chocolate-White Chocolate Chunk Cookie, 1 each	28	1
Oatmeal Raisin Pecan Cookie, 1 each	29	1
Coffee Coolatta® with 2% Milk, 16 ounce	49	0
Coffee Coolatta® with Cream, 16 ounce	48	0
Coffee Coolatta® with Milk, 16 ounce	49	0
Coffee Coolatta® with Skim Milk, 16 ounce	49	0
Iced Coffee with Skim Milk, 16 ounce	3	0
Iced Coffee with Skim Milk and Sugar, 16 ounce	15	0
Iced Coffee with Sugar, 16 ounce	13	0
Orange Mango Fruit Coolatta®, 16 ounce	69	<1
Strawberry Fruit Coolatta®, 16 ounce	68	1
Vanilla Bean Coolatta®, 16 ounce	73	0
Vanilla Chai, 10 ounce	37	0
Danish, Apple	36	0
Danish, Cheese	32	0
Danish, Cherry	34	0
Danish, Cinnamon	45	1
Danish, Strawberry Cheese	33	0
Munchkins, Butternut Cake, 3 each	25	<1
Munchkins, Cinnamon Cake, 4 each	30	<1
Munchkins, Coconut Cake, 3 each	23	<1
Munchkins, Glazed Cake, 3 each	27	0
Munchkins, Plain Cake, 4 each	22	<1
Munchkins, Powdered Cake, 4 each	29	<1
Munchkins, Sugared Cake, 4 each	28	<1
Munchkins, Toasted Coconut Cake, 3 each	24	<1
Munchkins, Glazed Chocolate Cake, 3 each	26	<1

	C	F
Munchkins, Glazed Yeast, 5 each	27	<1
Munchkins, Jelly Filled Yeast, 5 each	30	<1
Munchkins, Lemon Filled Yeast, 4 each	23	0
Munchkins, Sugar Raised Yeast, 7 each	26	<1
Donuts, Apple Crumb, 1 each	34	<1
Donuts, Apple N' Spice, 1 each	29	<1
Donuts, Bavarian Kreme, 1 each	30	<1
Donuts, Chocolate Iced Bismark, 1 each	50	<1
Donuts, Black Raspberry, 1 each	32	<1
Donuts, Blueberry Cake, 1 each	35	<1
Donuts, Blueberry Crumb, 1 each	36	<1
Donuts, Boston Kreme, 1 each	36	<1
Donuts, Bow Tie, 1 each	34	<1
Donuts, Butternut Cake Ring, 1 each	36	<1
Donuts, Chocolate Coconut Cake, 1 each	31	1
Donuts, Chocolate Frosted Cake, 1 each	38	<1
Donuts, Chocolate Frosted, 1 each	29	<1
Donuts, Chocolate Glazed Cake, 1 each	33	1
Donuts, Chocolate Kreme Filled, 1 each	35	<1
Donuts, Cinnamon Cake, 1 each	31	<1
Donuts, Coconut Cake, 1 each	33	<1
Donuts, Double Chocolate Cake, 1 each	37	2
Donuts, Dunkin' Donut, 1 each	25	<1

Einstein Bros. Bagels®

	C	F
Americano, large, 16 oz	0	0
Americano, regular, 8 oz	0	0
Ancho Lime Mayo, 1 tbsp	1	0
Ancho Lime Salsa, ¼ cup	3	0
Juice Box, Apple or Fruit Punch average, 1 box	27	NA
Asian Chicken w/ Peanut Sesame Half Flat Bread, 17.5 oz	152	8
Asian Sesame Dressing, 2 tbsp	16	0

	C	F
Bacon, Peppered, 3 slices	0	0
Bagel Croutons, ¼ cup	4	0
Bagel Mini Shtick Corn Meal, 1 each	38	1
Bagel Mini Shtick Sesame, 1 each	36	2
Bagel Shtick, Asiago, 1 each	72	2
Bagel Shtick, Cinnamon Sugar, 1 each	79	2
Bagel Shtick, Everything, 1 each	73	3
Bagel Shtick, Potato, 1 each	69	2
Bagel Shtick, Sesame, 1 each	75	5
Bagel, Asiago Cheese, 1 each	71	2
Bagel, Chocolate Chip, 1 each	76	3
Bagel, Chopped Garlic, 1 each	79	4
Bagel, Chopped Onion, 1 each	71	2
Bagel, Cinnamon Raisin Swirl, 1 each	78	2
Bagel, Cinnamon Sugar, 1 each	74	2
Bagel, Cranberry, 1 each	78	3
Bagel, Dark Pumpernickel, 1 each	68	3
Bagel, Egg, 1 each	69	2
Bagel, Everything, 1 each	75	2
Bagel, Honey Whole Wheat, 1 each	71	3
Bagel, Jalapeño, 1 each	71	2
Bagel, Lucky Green, 1 each	71	2
Bagel, Mango, 1 each	80	2
Bagel, Marble Rye, 1 each	73	3
Bagel, Nutty Banana, 1 each	74	2
Bagel, Plain, 1 each	71	2
Bagel, Poppy Dip'd, 1 each	74	2
Bagel, Potato, 1 each	69	2
Bagel, Power, 1 each	81	4
Bagel, Power Bagel with Peanut Butter, 1 each	92	7
Bagel, Pumpkin, 1 each	72	3
Bagel, Salt, 1 each	73	2
Bagel, Sesame Dip'd, 1 each	75	3
Bagel, Sun-Dried Tomato, 1 each	69	3
Bagel, Wild Blueberry, 1 each	77	3
Muffin Pumpkin Pecan, 5 oz	50	3
Black & White Cookie, 1	77	1

	C	F
Blueberry Figure 8, 1	48	1
Muffin Blueberry, 5 oz	57	2
Blueberry Scone with Icing, 1	64	2
Bros. Bistro w/ Rosemary Asiago Flat Bread, 13.1 oz	117	5
Brownie, 1	76	2
Cafe Latte, regular or nonfat, 12 oz	14	0
Cafe Latte, regular or nonfat, 16 oz	20	0
Cafe Latte, regular or nonfat, 20 oz	25	0
Cappuccino, regular or low fat average, 16 oz	17	0
Cappuccino, regular or low fat average, 20 oz	23	0
Cappuccino, regular, low fat or nonfat, 12 oz	9	0
Challah BBQ Chicken Sandwich, 1	52	2
Challah Club Mex, 1	47	2
Challah Cobbie, 1	45	4
Challah Deli Chicken Salad, 1	47	3
Challah Deli Egg Salad Sandwich, 1	45	2
Challah Deli Pastrami, 1	43	2
Challah Deli Roast Beef, 1	44	2
Challah Deli Smoked Turkey Sandwich, 1	44	2
Challah Deli Tuna Salad Sandwich, 1	42	2
Challah Deli Turkey Ham, 1	43	2
Challah Roasted Chicken & Smoked Gouda, 1	47	2
Challah Roll, 1 each	55	2
Cheese Pizza Focaccia, 1 each	75	3
Cheese, American, Cheddar, Provolone or Pepper Jack, 1 slice	0	0
Cherry Figure 8, 1	49	1
Chicago Bagel Dog (onion/no cheese), 1	78	2
Chicago Bagel Dog, Asiago, 1	78	2
Chicago Bagel Dog, Everything, 1	80	3
Chicago Chili Cheese Bagel Dog, 1	83	4
Chicken Chipotle Spinach Salad w/ Half Rosemary Asiago Flatbread, 15.8 oz	79	6
Chipotle BBQ Dressing, 2 tbsp	4	0
Muffin Banana Nut, 5 oz	59	3

	C	F
Chocolate Hazelnut Pastry, 1	51	3
Cinnamon Roll, 7.5 oz	118	4
Cinnamon Walnut Strudel, 1	63	3
Coffee, large, 20 oz	0	0
Coffee, medium, 16 oz	0	0
Coffee, regular, 12 oz	0	0
Coffee, regular decaffeinated, 12 oz	0	0
Cookie, Chocolate Chunk, Ginger. White Choc., or Oatmeal Raisin average, 4 oz	80	3
Cookie, Peanut Butter, 4 oz	66	2
Cookie, Sugar, 4 oz	73	1
Deli Chicken Salad on 12 Grain, 1	59	6
Deli Chicken Salad on Country White, 1	79	4
Deli Egg Salad on 12 Grain, 1	57	5
Deli Egg Salad on Country White, 1	77	3
Deli Ham on 12 Grain, 1	55	5
Deli Ham on Country White, 1	75	3
Deli Roast Beef on 12 Grain, 1	56	5
Deli Roast Beef on Country White, 1	76	3
Deli Smoked Turkey on 12 Grain, 1	56	5
Deli Smoked Turkey on Country White, 1	76	3
Deli Tuna Salad on 12 Grain, 1	54	5
Deli Tuna Salad on Country White, 1	74	3
Deli Turkey Pastrami on 12 Grain, 1	55	5
Deli Turkey Pastrami on Country White, 1	75	3
Dressing, Caesar, Horseradish Sauce, Harvest Chicken or Chicken/Tuna average, 2 tbsp	2	0
Dressing, Raspberry Vinaigrette, 2 tbsp	8	0
Egg Salad (Salad), 4 oz	5	0
Egg Salad Sandwich, 1	79	3
Egg, Homestyle Bacon, 1	74	2
Egg, Homestyle Ham, 1	74	2
Egg, Homestyle Sausage, 1	74	2
Egg, Original, 1	74	2
Egg, Salmon and Shmear, 1	82	3
Egg, Santa Fe, 1	78	2

	C	F		C	F
Espresso,Regular, 1.5 oz	0	0	Marinated Red Onions, 4 oz	9	2
Flat Bread, Peanut Sesame, 1 each	111	5	Mind Bageling Side, 3.5 oz	13	1
Flat Bread, Rosemary & Asiago, 1 each	92	3	Minute Maid Country Style OJ, 8 oz	27	0
			Minute Maid Orange, 8 oz	29	0
Fresh Fruit Cup, 8 oz	25	2	Minute Maid Orig. Style Lemonade, 8 oz	26	0
Fruitopia, Fruit Integration, 8 oz	29	0	
Fruitopia, Raspberry Psychic Lemonade, 8 oz	26	0	Minute Maid Premium OJ, 8 oz	27	0
			Mocha, regular or low fat, 12 oz	34	0
Fruitopia, Strawberry Passion Awareness, 8 oz	30	0	Mocha, regular or low fat, 16 oz	42	1
Fruitopia, Tangerine Wavelength, 8 oz	29	0	Mocha, regular or low fat, 20 oz	56	1
Fruitopia, The Grape Beyond, 8 oz	27	0	Muffin Lemon Poppyseed low fat, 5 oz	69	1
Half & Half, 2 tbsp	1	NA	Mr. Pibb, 8 oz	26	0
Ham, 1	74	3	Mustard: Deli, Dijon, or Yellow, 1 tsp	0	0
Handle Bar, 1	113	9	Nestea Peach Iced Tea, 8 oz	21	0
Harvest Chicken Salad, 1	81	4	Nestea Raspberry Iced Tea, 8 oz	21	0
Harvest Chicken w/ Rosemary & Asiago Flat Bread, 12.5 oz	103	5	Nestea Southern Style Iced Tea, 8 oz	33	0
Hi C Fruit Punch, 8 oz	28	0	New York Lox & Bagels, 1	79	3
Hi C Grape, 8 oz	28	0	Odwalla Fresh Squeezed OJ, 10 oz	34	2
Hi C Light Fruit Punch, Lemon-lime, Orange, Pink Lemonade, 8 oz	0	0	On Top Reduced Fat Topping, 2 tbsp	2	0
			Pecan Pie Pastry, 1	47	2
Hi C Orange, 8 oz	30	0	Pepperoni Pizza Focaccia	76	3
Hi C Pink Lemonade, 8 oz	25	0	Pound Cake, Lemon Iced	74	0
Holey Cow, 1	77	3	Pound Cake, Marble	57	1
Honey Chipotle Dressing, 2 tbsp	12	0	Pull-Apart Cinnamon Bun w/Icing	64	2
Honey Mustard, 2 tbsp	12	0	Pull-Apart Sticky Bun	77	3
Hot Chocolate, regular, 12 oz	39	0	Muffin Morning Harvest	69	4
Hummus & Feta, 1	89	5	Raspberry Low Fat Scone	74	2
Hummus, Retail, 2 oz	9	2	Raspberry Mustard	7	0
Iced Americano, 8 oz	0	0	Rice Krispy Bars	83	1
Iced Coffee, 12 oz	0	0	Roast Beef	76	3
Iced Latte, regular or nonfat, 16 oz	12	0	Roasted Chicken Caesar w/Rosemary & Asiago Flat Bread	86	4
Iced Mocha, regular or low fat, 16 oz	33	0	Roasted Corn Salad	13	4
Iced Tea, unsweetened, 8 oz	0	0	Roll-Up Albuquerque Turkey	81	5
Light Whipped Cream, 2 tbsp	2	0	Roll-Up Thai Vegetable	97	5
Muffin Chocolate Chip, 2 oz	67	0	Roll-Up Thai Vegetable w/Chicken	99	4
Lower Fat Hot Chocolate, regular, 12 oz	39	0	Root Beer, Stewart's	40	0
Low fat 2% Milk, 8 oz	12	0	Skim Milk	15	0
Margherita Focaccia, 1 each	76	3	Small Caesar Side	12	1

	C	F
Smoked Salmon, Port Chatham	2	0
Smoked Salmon, Sea Specialties	1	0
Smoked Turkey	75	3
Smoothie, Mocha	98	0
Soups, Chicken & Wild Rice, large	30	3
Soups, Chicken & Wild Rice, small	18	2
Soups, Chicken Noodle, large	30	4
Soups, Chicken Noodle, small	19	2
Soups, Cream of Potato, large	35	5
Soups, Cream of Potato, small	23	3
Soups, Red Beans & Rice, large	40	9
Soups, Red Beans & Rice, small	26	6
Soups, Turkey Chili w/Beans, large	28	3
Soups, Turkey Chili w/Beans, small	20	2
Soups, Vegetarian Black Bean, large	34	10
Soups, Vegetarian Black Bean, small	23	7
Soups, Zesty Lentil, large	34	11
Soups, Zesty Lentil, small	20	7
Spreads, Apricot, Grape or Strawberry	19	0
Spreads, Honey Butter or Peanut Butter	8	0
Sprite	26	0
Sweet Roasted Walnuts	7	1
Sweetie Pie	163	1.5
Swiss Cheese	1	0
Syrup, Almond	23	0
Syrup, Hazelnut	20	0
Syrup, Premium, Sugar Free Caramel or Vanilla	0	0
Syrup, Raspberry	20	0
Syrup, Vanilla	19	0
Tasty Turkey	78	3
The Veg Out	77	3
Thousand Island	5	0
Traditional Potato Salad	21	2
Tuna Salad	77	3
Tuna Salad	3	0
Turkey Pastrami Deli	76	3
Turkey Pastrami Rueben Deli	83	4
Ultimate Toasted Cheese w/ Tomato on 12 Grain	53	4

	C	F
Ultimate Toasted Cheese w/ Tomato on Country White	73	2
Wasabi Oriental Dressing	5	0
Wasabi Salmon Spinach Salad w/ Half Peanut Sesame Flatbread	84	6
Whipped Blueberry	6	0
Whipped Cappuccino	4	0
Whipped Garden Vegetable	2	0
Whipped Honey Almond Red.	5	0
Whipped Jalapeño Salsa	3	0
Whipped Maple Raisin Walnut	4	0
Whipped Onion and Chive	2	0
Whipped Plain	1	0
Whipped Plain Reduced Fat	2	0
Whipped Smoked Salmon	3	0
Whipped Strawberry	5	0
Whipped Sundried Tomato & Basil	2	0
Whole Kosher Pickle	1	1

El Pollo Loco®

	C	F
Flame Grilled Chicken Breast w/skin, 1 serving	0	
Flame Grilled Chicken Leg, 1 serving	0	
Flame Grilled Chicken Thigh, 1 serving	0	
Flame Grilled Chicken Wing, 1 serving	0	
Burritos, Chicken Guacamole, 1 serving	59	
Burritos, Classic BRC, 1 serving	79	
Burritos, Classic Chicken Lovers, 1 serving	55	
Burritos, Classic Chicken, 1 serving	81	
Burritos, Classic Spicy Chicken, 1 serving	64	
Burritos, Grilled Signature, Grilled Fiesta, 1 serving	91	
Burritos, Grilled Signature, Twice Grilled, 1 serving	62	
Burritos, Grilled Signature, Ultimate Chicken, 1 serving	84	
Bowls, Chicken Caesar Salad, 1 serving	47	
Bowls, Pollo, 1 serving	84	

	C	F
Loco Favorites, Cheese Quesadilla, 1 serving	51	
Loco Favorites, Chicken Nachos, 1 serving	90	
Loco Favorites, Chicken Quesadilla, 1 serving	53	
Loco Favorites, Chicken Soft Taco, 1 serving	18	
Loco Favorites, Chicken Taquitos, 1 serving	43	
Loco Favorites, Taco el Carbon, 1 serving	18	
Salads, w/ dressing, Chicken Caesar, 1 serving	17	
Salads, w/ dressing, Chicken Fiesta, 1 serving	29	
Salads, w/ dressing, Chicken Monterray, 1 serving	17	
Salads, w/ dressing, Chicken Tostada, 1 serving	83	
Salads, w/ dressing, Tostada no shell, 1 serving	42	
Salads, w/ dressing, Tamales, 1 Tamale	21	
Side Dishes, Coleslaw, 5 oz	12	
Side Dishes, Corn Cobette, 3 oz	10	
Side Dishes, French Fries, 5.5 oz	61	
Side Dishes, Fresh Vegetables, 4 oz	6	
Side Dishes, Garden Salad, 4.8 oz	8	
Side Dishes, Pinto Beans, 6 oz	24	
Side Dishes, Spanish Rice, 4 oz	33	
Side Dishes, Tortilla Chips, small, 2 oz	34	
Tortillas, 6" corn, 6", 3 oz	42	
Tortillas, 6 ½" flour, 3 oz	48	
Dressings, Creamy Chipotle, 1 serving	3	
Dressings, Creamy Cilantro, 1 serving	1	
Dressings, Guacamole, 1.7 oz	5	
Dressings, Jalopeño Hot Sauce, 0.3 oz pkt	0	
Dressings, Sour Cream, 1 serving	2	
Salsa, Avocado, 1 serving	1	
Salsa, Chipotle, House, 1 serving	1	

	C	F
Salsa, Pico de Gallo, 1 serving	1	
Desserts, Churro, 1 churro	24	
Desserts, Flan, 5.5 oz	43	
Desserts, Soft Serve, regular, 5.0 oz	30	

El Torito ®

	C	F
Frijoles de la Olla, 1 (4) oz serving	29	8
Grilled Chicken Quesadilla Lite, 1 serving	48	4
Grilled Soft Chicken Tacos (Special Request)—includes rice and frijoles	51	4
Mexican-Style Rice, 1 (4 oz) serving	32	0
Sonora Burrito Lite, 1 serving	63	8
Spinach Enchiladas (Special Request), 1 serving	44	7

Fresh Choice ®

BAKERY / BREADS

	C	F
Almond Poppyseed, 1 piece	41	1
Apple Cinnamon, 1 piece	42	2
Apple Cranberry Crunch, 1 piece	51	2
Apple Honey Bran, 1 piece	53	2
Apricot Almond, 1 piece	41	1
Banana Nut, 1 piece	39	2
Banana Pineapple, 1 piece	43	1
Banana Raspberry, 1 piece	45	1
Blueberry, 1 piece	35	1
Blueberry Orange, 1 piece	41	1
Breadsticks, 1 piece	31	0
Brownie Chip, 1 piece	47	2
Chocolate Almond, 1 piece	37	2
Chocolate Cheesecake Swirl, 1 piece	44	1
Chocolate Coconut, 1 piece	38	1
Chocolate Covered Banana, 1 piece	49	2
Chocolate Mint Chip, 1 piece	40	1
Chocolate Orange, 1 piece	43	2
Chocolate Peanut Crunch, 1 piece	42	2
Chocolate Raspberry, 1 piece	44	2
Corn, 1 piece	34	0

	C	F
Country Herb Biscuit, 1 Biscuit	36	0
Cranberry Orange, 1 piece	45	2
Dutch Apple Crunch, 1 piece	50	2
Fresh Banana, 1 piece	44	1
German Chocolate, 1 piece	49	2
Harvest Bread, 2 oz serving	22	1
Honey Peach, 1 piece	48	1
Lemon Poppyseed, 1 piece	39	1
Orange Peach, 1 piece	43	1
Peach Cinnamon, 1 piece	35	1
Peach Cinnamon Crunch, 1 piece	45	2
Peach Melba, 1 piece	39	1
Pineapple Apricot, 1 piece	45	1
Pineapple Nut, 1 piece	38	1
Pumpkin Craisin Crunch, 1 piece	49	2
Pumpkin Spice, 1 piece	47	1
Raspberry Orange, 1 piece	40	1
Raspberry Peach, 1 piece	31	1
Santa Fe Corn, 1 piece	37	0
Sourdough Bread, 2 oz serving	25	0
Strawberry Banana, 1 piece	46	1
Zucchini, Carrot and Raisin, 1 piece	42	1

DESSERTS

	C	F
Apple Caramel Cobbler Cake, 1 piece	33	1
Chocolate Pudding, ½ cup	30	1
Double Chocolate Cake, ½ cup	38	1
German Chocolate Cake, ½ cup	41	1
Lemon Pudding Cake, 1 piece	31	0
Old-Fashioned Bread Pudding, 1 piece	23	1
Orange Sicle Cake, 1 piece	31	0
Peach Cobbler Cake, 1 piece	31	1
Pina Colada Bread Pudding, 1 serving	22	1
Smore Cake, 1 piece	21	1
Tapioca Pudding, ½ cup	23	0
Triple Decadence Brownie, 1 brownie	24	1
Soft Serve, Chocolate, ½ cup	27	1
Soft Serve, Vanilla, ½ cup	26	0

PASTAS

	C	F
Alfredo, 2 oz	5	0
Bolognese with Meatball, 2 oz	4	1
Broccoli Cheddar with Ham, 2 oz	4	0
Broccoli with Cheese, 2 oz	4	0
Chicken Cacciatore, 2 oz	10	0
Clam and Mushroom, 2 oz	4	0
Creamy Lemon Piccata, 2 oz	35	2
Creamy Pesto, 2 oz	5	0
Creamy Sundried Tomato Pesto, 2 oz	5	0
Garden Marinara, 2 oz	4	1
Mushroom Stroganoff, 2 oz	4	0
Plain, ½ cup	21	1
Ragin Cajun Gumbo with Andouille, 2 oz	9	2
Santa Fe Red with Chicken, 2 oz	6	1
Tuscany Cream, 2 oz	4	0

PIZZAS

	C	F
Cheese, 1 slice	19	1
Chicken Garlic Alfredo, 1 slice	19	1
Fresh Tomato Basil, 1 slice	19	1
Greek, 1 slice	20	1
Mediterranean, 1 slice	20	1
Pepperoni, 1 slice	19	1
Pesto Ranch with Smoked Bacon, 1 slice	19	1
Vegetarian, 1 slice	20	1

PREPARED SALADS

	C	F
Almond Chicken Pasta, ½ cup	16	1
Antipasto, ½ cup	15	1
Artichoke and Bowite Pasta, ½ cup	16	1
Asian Broccoli Slaw, ½ cup	6	2
Baked Potato, ½ cup	14	1
Basil Aioli with Wild Rice, ½ cup	21	1
Caesar Pasta, ½ cup	15	1
Cavatappi Pesto, ½ cup	25	1
Chicken Basil Aioli, ½ cup	22	1
Chicken Caesar Mexicali, ½ cup	17	2
Chicken Cobb, ½ cup	8	2
Chicken Pesto Penne, ½ cup	12	1

	C	F
Chinese Chicken, ½ cup	11	3
Classic Picnic Slaw, ½ cup	3	1
Country Picnic Potato, ½ cup	15	1
Creamy Citrus Slaw, ½ cup	6	1
Creamy Dill Potato, ½ cup	18	1
Creamy Peanut Slaw, ½ cup	5	1
Crisp Apple Pineapple, ½ cup	20	2
Fresh Vegetable Medley, ½ cup	4	1
Ginger Soy Long Noodle, ½ cup	21	1
Greek Goddess Medley, ½ cup	11	1
Greek Salad, ½ cup	21	2
Italian Tomato and Cucumber, ½ cup	4	1
Italian Vegetable Medley, ½ cup	4	1
Lemon Garlic Pasta, ½ cup	17	1
Mardi Gras Cajun Pasta, ½ cup	15	2
Marinated Cucumber, ½ cup	5	1
Mom's Mac, ½ cup	19	1
Palermo Pasta, ½ cup	17	1
Pasta Pomodoro, ½ cup	17	1
Peppercorn Ranch Pasta, ½ cup	15	1
Pina Colada Slaw, ½ cup	4	1
Radiatore Pasta, ½ cup	16	1
Raspberry and Walnut with Chicken, ½ cup	12	1
Rice with Artichoke, ½ cup	16	1
Roasted Red Potato, ½ cup	17	1
Roasted Vegetable, ½ cup	21	2
Seafood Pasta, ½ cup	16	1
Shrimp and Bowtie, ½ cup	11	1
Smashed Potato, ½ cup	25	2
Spinach Dijon, ½ cup	11	2
Summer Garden Pasta, ½ cup	12	2
Sweet and Sour Broccoli, ½ cup	11	2
Thai Shredded Slaw, ½ cup	8	1
Thai Shrimp and Snow Pea, ½ cup	17	1
Tuna Tarragon, ½ cup	16	1
Waldorf Lite, ½ cup	19	2

SALAD DRESSINGS

	C	F
1000 Island, 2 oz	4	0
Balsamic Vinegarette, 2 oz	8	0
Bleu Cheese, 2 oz	2	0
Caesar, 2 oz	2	0
Chinese Chicken Dressing, 2 oz	14	0
French, fat free, 2 oz	16	0
Honey Dijon, fat free, 2 oz	13	0
Italian, fat free, 2 oz	0	0
Parmesan Peppercorn, 2 oz	2	0
Ranch, 2 oz	2	0
Ranch, fat free, 2 oz	6	0

SOUPS

	C	F
Baked Potato, 1 cup	21	2
Broccoli Cheddar, 1 cup	15	2
Carrot Ginger, 1 cup	20	5
Chile Verde, 1 cup	21	6
Confetti Bean Chili, 1 cup	28	8
Cream of Asparagus, 1 cup	16	1
Cream of Broccoli, 1 cup	12	2
Cream of Mushroom, 1 cup	14	1
Creamy Tomato Bisque, 1 cup	21	1
Fall Harvest Squash, 1 cup	20	3
Fettucine Chicken Noodle, 1 cup	18	2
Firehouse Chili, 1 cup	32	8
French Onion, 1 cup	16	2
Grandma's Chicken & Dumplings, 1 cup	17	1
Green Chili and Corn Chowder, 1 cup	26	2
Harvest Vegetable, 1 cup	20	4
Hearty Vegetable, 1 cup	9	2
Mushroom Bean and Barley, 1 cup	29	7
Navy Bean and Ham, 1 cup	36	8
New England Clam Chowder, 1 cup	26	1
New Orleans Vegetarian Gumbo, 1 cup	18	3
Potato Cheddar, 1 cup	22	1
Potato Leek, 1 cup	27	2
Red Bean Chili, 1 cup	41	11
Roasted Sirloin Chili, 1 cup	29	6
San Jose Chicken Chili, 1 cup	29	6
Savory Bean, 1 cup	27	6

	C	F
Smoke House Potato Cheddar, 1 cup	22	1
Southern Lentil, 1 cup	20	6
Southwestern Black Bean with Andouille, 1 cup	20	5
Southwestern Corn Chowder, 1 cup	24	2
Spicy Meatball, 1 cup	16	2
Spicy Texas Chili Con Carne, 1 cup	27	7
Split Pea with Ham, 1 cup	18	6
Summer Squash, 1 cup	7	2
Texas Chicken Tortilla, 1 cup	20	3
Thai Chicken Coconut, 1 cup	22	1
Turkey and Wild Rice, 1 cup	14	1
Turkey Chili, low fat, 1 cup	78	8
Turkey Chili, regular, 1 cup	33	8
Turkey Gumbo, 1 cup	19	3
Turkey Rice, 1 cup	12	1
Tuscan Tortellini Minestrone, 1 cup	24	5
Tuscan White Bean and Vegetable, 1 cup	26	6
Vegetable Barley, 1 cup	25	4
Vegetable Minestrone, 1 cup	16	3
Vegetarian Vegetable, 1 cup	14	3
Yankee Pot Roast Soup, 1 cup	20	2

SPECIALTY SALADS

	C	F
Azteca Ensalada, 1 cup	8	2
Caribbean Chicken Salad, 1 cup	19	4
Classic Caesar Salad, 1 cup	8	1
Classic Shrimp Louie Salad, 1 cup	5	1
Club Sandwich, 1 cup	5	2
Cool Raspberry Crunch, 1 cup	13	2
Raspberry and Walnut, 1 cup	12	1
Southern Fried Chicken, 1 cup	12	3
Spicy Buffalo Chicken, 1 cup	5	2
Szechuan Beef, 1 cup	13	2

Friendly's ®

WRAPS

	C	F
Buffalo Chicken Sandwich Wrap (1)	75	4
Crispy Chicken Sandwich Wrap (1)	86	5
Oriental Chicken Sandwich Wrap (1)	135	10

	C	F
French Fries, 6 oz	39	4

Godfather's Pizza®

	C	F
Golden, Cheese: medium, ⅛ pizza, 1 slice	26	
Golden, Cheese: large, ⅒ pizza, 1 slice	28	
Golden, Combo: medium, ⅛ pizza, 1 slice	27	
Golden, Combo: large, ⅒ pizza, 1 slice	30	
Original, Cheese: Mini, 14 pizzas, 1 slice	20	
Original, Cheese: medium, ⅛ pizza, 1 slice	34	
Original, Cheese: Jumbo, ⅒ pizza, 1 slice	53	
Original, Combo: Mini, 14 pizzas, 1 slice	21	
Original: medium, ⅛ pizza, 1 slice	36	
Original: Jumbo, ⅒ pizza, 1 slice	57	
Thin, Cheese: medium, ⅛ pizza, 1 slice	19	
Thin, Cheese: large, ⅒ pizza, 1 slice	19	
Thin, Combo: medium, ⅛ pizza, 1 slice	21	
Thin, Combo: large, ⅒ pizza, 1 slice	21	
Sides: Breadstick, 1 stick	14	
Sides: Cheesestick, ⅙ whole, 1 piece	18	
Sides: Chocolate Chip Cookie, 1 slice	30	
Sides: Potato Wedges, 4 oz	24	

Great Harvest Bread Co ®

BREADS

	C	F
Apple Crunch Bread, 1 slice	23	3
Challa Bread, 1 slice	23	2
Cheddar Garlic Bread, 1 slice	16	2
Cheddar Garlic Low Carb Bread, 1 slice	7	1
Cherry Walnut Bread, 1 slice	24	2
Cinnamon Chip Bread (Wheat Flour), 1 slice	24	3

	C	F
Cinnamon Chip Low Carb Bread, 1 slice	9	2
Cinnamon Raisin Low Carb Bread, 1 slice	10	2
Cinnamon Raisin Walnut Bread, 1 slice	23	3
Cinnamon Swirl Bread, 1 slice	26	3
Cracked Pepper Parmesan Bread, 1 slice	19	9
Cranberry Orange Bread, 1 slice	25	3
Dakota Bread, 1 slice	21	3
Dakota Low Carb Bread, 1 slice	8	2
Flax Oat Bran Bread, 1 slice	21	4
High Country Crunch Low Carb Bread, 1 slice	9	2
Honey Whole Wheat Bread, 1 slice	23	3
Irish Soda Bread, 1 slice	24	2
Nine Grain Bread, 1 slice	23	3
Oat Bran Bread, 1 slice	21	3
Oatmeal Poppyseed Bread, 1 slice	23	3
Oregon Herb Bread, 1 slice	23	3
Pumpkin Swirl Bread, 1 slice	22	2
Raisin Bread, 1 slice	24	2
Red, White and Blueberry Bread, 1 slice	25	<1
Spelt Bread, 1 slice	27	2
Spinach Feta Bread, 1 slice	16	1
Sunflower Bread, 1 slice	22	3
Sunflower Millet Bread, 1 slice	23	3
White Bread, 1 slice	23	<1
White Chocolate Cherry Swirl Bread, 1 slice	27	<1
Whole Grain Goodness Bread, 1 slice	21	3
Whole Grain Low Carb Bread, 1 slice	8	2

BARS & COOKIES

	C	F
Savannah Bars, 1 bar	87	7
Chocolate Chip Oatmeal Walnut Cookie, 1 cookie	64	5
Raisin Oatmeal Cookie, 1 cookie	72	5

MUFFINS, ROLLS & SCONES

	C	F
Berry Oat Bran Muffin, 1 muffin	57	7
Cinnamon Roll (no frosting), 1 roll	105	9
Berry Cream Cheese Scone, 1 scone	40	1
Cinnamon Chip Scone, 1 scone	41	<1

Hibachi-San Japanese Grill ®

ENTREES

	C	F
Sauteed Vegetables entrée, (1) 5 oz serving	10	1
Shiromi Chicken entrée, (1) 4oz serving	0	0
Teriyaki Beef entrée, (1) 4 oz serving	7	1
Teriyaki Chicken entrée, (1) 4 oz serving	4	2

APPETIZERS

	C	F
Assorted Sushi box - 6 rolls	51	2
California Roll box - 8 rolls	75	6
Spicy Tuna Roll box - 10 rolls	67	3
Sunrise Roll box - 8 rolls	69	2
Vegetable Roll box - 10 rolls	79	5

MISCELLANEOUS

	C	F
Fried Rice, (1) 8 oz order	77	3
Lo Mein Noodles, (1) 6 oz order	42	5
Steamed Rice, (1) 6 oz order	65	0
Spicy Honey Sauce, 3 oz	50	0
Teriyaki Sauce, 3 oz	20	0
Udon Noodle Soup with Seaweed and Broth, 1 order	78	5

Hometown Buffet ®

BREADS / MUFFINS / ROLLS

	C	F
Biscuits, 1 biscuit	24	1
Biscuits, Cheese Garlic, 1 biscuit	22	<1
Breadsticks, 1 breadstick	21	1
Buns, Hot Dog, 1 bun	22	1
Buns, Sandwich, 1 bun	22	1
Caramel Rolls, 1 roll	24	1
Cinnamon Bread, 1 slice	10	0
Cinnamon Rolls, Glazed, 1 roll	31	<1
Corn Muffins, 1 muffin	40	0
Cornbread, Plain, 1 piece	23	0
Dinner Rolls, Savory, 1 roll	20	1

	C	F
Dinner Rolls, Wheat, 1 roll	18	1
Dinner Rolls, White, 1 roll	20	1
Muffin, Blueberry (1)	38	<1
Muffin, English, ½ muffin	13	<1

BREAKFAST

	C	F
Corned Beef Hash, 1 spoonful	11	3
Denver Scrambled Eggs, 1 spoonful	2	0
Eggs Benedict, 1 egg	15	1
Eggs, Hard-Cooked, Diced, 1 spoonful	0	0
Eggs, Poached, 1 egg	0	0
Eggs, Scrambled, 1 spoonful	<1	0
French Toast, 1 slice	24	<1
Grits, 1 ladle	16	0
Oatmeal, 1 ladle	13	2
Pancakes, (1)	19	<1
Quiche, Breakfast, 1 spoonful	12	0
Waffles, 1 waffle	19	<1

ENTREES / CHICKEN

	C	F
Chicken and Dumplings, 1 spoonful	24	<1
Chicken Cacciatore, 1 spoonful	3	<1
Chicken Marsala, 1 piece	3	0
Chicken Pot Pie, Crustless, 1 spoonful	5	0
Chicken, Hand-Breaded, Fried (1) Breast	3	0
Chicken, Hand-Breaded, Fried (1) Drumstick	2	0
Chicken, Hand-Breaded, Fried (1) Thigh	4	0
Chicken, Traditional Baked (1) Breast	0	0
Chicken, Traditional Baked (1) Drumstick	0	0
Chicken, Traditional Baked (1) Thigh	0	0
Orange Chicken, 1 spoonful	24	0
Smothered Chicken, 1 piece	3	0
Teriyaki Chicken Wings (1) Drummie	2	0
Teriyaki Chicken Wings (1) Wing	2	0

ENTREES / BEEF

	C	F
BBQ Beef Ribs, 1 order	7	0
BBQ Smoked Sausage, 1 spoonful	9	<1
Beef Brisket, Carved, 3 oz	1	0
Beef Liver and Onions, 1 piece	4	0
Beef Patties with Mushroom Gravy, 1 patty	2	0
Hamburger Patties, 1 patty	0	0
Italian Meatballs with Sauce, 1 meatball	2	0
Meatloaf, 1 piece	9	0
Pot Roast Vegetables with gravy, 4 oz	13	2
Pot Roast with gravy, 4 oz	1	0
Roast Beef, Carved, 3 oz	0	0

ENTREES / OTHER

	C	F
Cheese Enchiladas, 1 enchilada	13	1
Fish Patties, 1 piece	13	0
Fish, Baked, 1 piece	0	0
Fish, Fried, 1 piece	9	0
Ham, Carved, 3 oz	0	0
Hot Dogs, Turkey (1)	2	0
Hot Wings - Drummies, (1)	0	0
Hot Wings - Wing, (1)	0	0
Italian Sausage with Vegetables, 1 link plus veggies	3	<1
Mini Corn Dogs, 1 piece	6	0
Pizza, Cheese, 1 slice	6	0
Pizza, Deep Dish - Three Cheese, (1) Slice	10	<1
Pizza, Deep Dish - Pepperoni & Sausage, (1) Slice	13	<1
Pork Loin, Peppered, Carved, 3 oz	0	0
Roast Turkey, Carved, 3 oz	0	0
Salmon Filet, Carved, 3 oz	0	0
Shrimp, Fried, 6 pieces	11	0
Smoked Sausage & Sauerkraut (Sauerkraut Only), 1 spoonful	1	0
Smoked Sausage & Sauerkraut (Sausage Only), 1 link	2	0
Taco Meat, Beef, 1 ladle	3	0
Taco Shells, 1 shell	7	0
Tortilla, Flour 1 tortilla	20	1

	C	F
Vegetable Stir-Fry, 1 spoonful	6	2

FRUIT

	C	F
Cantaloupe, 1 spoonful	6	<1
Grapes, 1 spoonful	15	<1
Honeydew, 1 spoonful	8	<1
Pineapple, 1 spoonful	10	1
Raisins, 1 spoonful	10	<1
Strawberries, 1 spoonful	6	1
Watermelon, 1 spoonful	6	0

VEGETABLES

	C	F
Asparagus, Herbed, 1 spoonful	4	1
Broccoli, Herbed, 1 spoonful	5	3
Brussel Sprouts, Herbed, 1 spoonful	8	2
Cabbage, German Boiled, 1 spoonful	3	1
Cabbage, Green, 1 spoonful	3	1
Carrots, Julienne, 1 spoonful	1	0
Carrots, Steamed, 1 spoonful	9	3
Cauliflower, Herbed, 1 spoonful	4	2
Chesapeake Corn, 1 spoonful	13	2
Collard Greens with Bacon, 1 spoonful	2	1
Corn, Steamed, 1 spoonful	21	2
Green Bean Casserole, 1 spoonful	9	2
Green Beans El Greco, 1 spoonful	5	2
Green Beans, 1 spoonful	3	1
Green Beans, Herbed, 1 spoonful	6	2
Green Peppers, sauteed, 1 spoonful	4	<1
Italian-Style Green Beans with Bacon, 1 spoonful	5	2
Joe's Cracked Pepper Green Beans, 1 spoonful	5	2
Lima Beans, Herbed, 1 spoonful	16	5
Lima Beans, Steamed, 1 spoonful	19	4
Marinated Vegetables, 1 spoonful	6	1
Montreal Vegetable Medley, 1 spoonful	3	1
Peas, 1 spoonful	2	1
Spinach Leaves, 1 cup	1	<1
Spinach Marie, 1 spoonful	8	1
Spring Mix, 1 cup	1	1

	C	F
Squash, Winter, 1 spoonful	18	1
Sweet Potatoes, Baked, 1 potato	47	6
Turnip Greens with Bacon, 1 spoonful	2	1
Yams, Candied, 1 spoonful	30	1
Zucchini, Sauteed, 1 spoonful	3	1

SOUPS

	C	F
Chicken Noodle Soup, 1 ladle	7	<1
Chicken Rice Soup, 1 ladle	8	<1
Chili Bean Soup, 1 ladle	9	1
Corn Chowder, 1 ladle	15	1
Cream of Broccoli Soup, 1 ladle	5	1
Navy Bean Soup with Ham, 1 ladle	10	4
New England Clam Chowder, 1 ladle	9	0
Potato Cheese Soup, 1 ladle	11	1

SALADS

	C	F
BLT Salad, 1 spoonful	3	<1
Broccoli Apple Salad, 1 spoonful	13	2
Caesar Salad, 1 cup	5	1
California Coleslaw, 1 spoonful	22	1
Carrot and Raisin Salad, 1 spoonful	18	2
Chicken Pasta Salad, 1 spoonful	11	1
Coleslaw, Creamy, 1 spoonful	12	2
Cucumber Tomato Salad, 1 spoonful	6	1
Greek Salad, 1 spoonful	11	1
Macaroni Vegetable Salad, 1 spoonful	20	1
Pea Salad, Creamy, 1 spoonful	11	4
Potato Salad, 1 spoonful	14	1
Potato Salad, Dilled, 1 spoonful	9	1
Seafood Salad, 1 spoonful	16	1
Seven-Layer Salad, 1 spoonful	4	1
Sicilian Pasta Salad, 1 spoonful	15	2
Strawberry-Banana Salad, 1 spoonful	16	2
Strawberry-Peach-Banana Salad, 1 spoonful	20	1
Tarragon Potato Salad, 1 spoonful	13	1
Three-Bean Salad, 1 spoonful	12	3
Tossed Green Salad, 1 cup	1	1
Waldorf Salad, 1 spoonful	12	1

	C	F
Whipped Pineapple and Banana Salad, 1 spoonful	33	0
DRESSINGS		
Italian Dressing, 1 ladle	5	0
Italian Dressing, Creamy, 1 ladle	3	0
Italian Dressing, Low Fat, 1 ladle	2	0
Ranch Dressing, 1 ladle	1	0
Ranch Dressing, Reduced Fat, 1 ladle	2	0
Thousand Island Dressing, 1 ladle	6	0
SAUCES & GRAVY		
Au Jus Sauce, 1 ladle	0	0
Cheese Sauce, Creamy, 1 ladle	9	0
Cocktail Sauce, 1 ladle	8	0
Cranberry Sauce, 1 ladle	12	0
Gravy, Beef, 1 ladle	2	0
Gravy, Chicken, 1 ladle	5	0
Gravy, Country, 1 ladle	12	0
Gravy, Roasted Pork, 1 ladle	3	0
Gravy, Turkey, 1 ladle	2	0
Hollandaise Sauce, 1 ladle	3	0
Horseradish Sauce, 1 ladle	2	0
Hot Sauce, 1 teaspoon	0	0
Marinara Sauce, 1 ladle	6	2
Meat Sauce, 1 ladle	4	<1
Soy Sauce, 1 teaspoon	<1	0
Tabasco Sauce, 1 teaspoon	0	0
Tartar Sauce, 1 ladle	4	0
POTATOES, PASTA, RICE		
French Fries, 22 fries	24	2
Fried Rice with Ham, 1 spoonful	23	1
FunE Chips, 1 spoonful	12	0
Jasmine Rice, 1 spoonful	28	0
Macaroni and Cheese, 1 spoonful	26	<1
Mostaciolli, 1 spoonful	13	1
Oriental Pasta, 1 spoonful	11	2
Potatoes, Baked, 1 potato	39	3
Potatoes, Cowboy-Grilled, 1 spoonful	15	2
Potatoes, Hash Brown Patties, 1 patty	11	1

	C	F
Potatoes, Hash Browns, 1 spoonful	13	1
Potatoes, JoJo, 6 pieces	18	2
Potatoes, Mashed, 1 spoonful	30	3
Potatoes, O'Brien, 1 spoonful	16	2
Potatoes, Red, 1 spoonful	18	2
Scalloped Potatoes with Ham, 1 spoonful	18	1
Scalloped Potatoes, 1 spoonful	19	1
Scalloped Potatoes, Loaded, 1 spoonful	20	1
Spaghetti, 1 spoonful	19	1
Spanish Rice, 1 spoonful	9	1
White Rice, 1 spoonful	22	<1
Wild Rice Vegetable Pilaf, 1 spoonful	17	<1
SIDES		
Bacon, 1 slice	0	0
Baked Beans, 1 spoonful	29	4
Black Olives, Sliced, 1 spoonful	1	<1
Cherry Peppers, 1 spoonful	1	0
Cherry Tomatoes, 1 tomato	1	0
Chinese Chicken Livers, 1 spoonful	17	1
Corn on the Cob, 1 piece	16	1
Cucumbers, (1) Slice	<1	0
Jalapeno Peppers, 1 spoonful	<1	0
Lettuce, shredded, ¼ cup	0	0
Mushrooms, Sauteed, 1 spoonful	2	<1
Mushrooms, Sliced, 1 spoonful	<1	0
Onions, Diced, 1 spoonful	2	0
Onions, Sauteed, 1 spoonful	5	<1
Pepperoncini Peppers, 1 spoonful	<1	0
Pickled Beets, 1 spoonful	25	2
Pickles, sliced, 1 spoonful	<1	0
Pinto Beans with Ham, 1 spoonful	21	7
Prunes, Stewed, 1 spoonful	28	2
Red Beans with Ham, 1 spoonful	18	7
Red Onions, Sliced, 1 ring	<1	0
Sausage Links, 1 link	0	0
Tomatoes, sliced or diced, 1 spoonful	<1	0

TOPPINGS	C	F
Apple Topping, 1 ladle	14	1
Bacon Bits, Imitation, 1 spoonful	2	<1
Bacon Bits, Real, 1 spoonful	0	0
Blueberry Syrup, 1 ladle	63	0
Brown Sugar, 1 tablespoon	9	0
Butterfinger Pieces, 1 spoonful	11	0
Butterscotch Topping, 1 pump	56	0
Cheese, Feta, 1 spoonful	<1	0
Cheese, Grated Parmesan, 1 spoonful	0	0
Cheese, Imitation, Shredded, 1 spoonful	2	0
Cheese, Shredded Cheddar, 1 spoonful	0	0
Chocolate Chips, 1 spoonful	10	0
Chocolate Syrup, 1 pump	21	0
Chow Mein Noodles, 1 spoonful	4	<1
Gummy Bears, 9 pieces	15	0
Gummy Worms, 3 pieces	14	0
Honey Nut Topping, 1 spoonful	7	2
Hot Fudge Topping, 1 pump	23	0
Hydrox Cookies, Crushed, 1 spoonful	6	0
Malted Milk Balls, Ground, 1 spoonful	11	0
Maple Syrup, 1 ladle	47	0
Nestle Crunch Pieces, 1 spoonful	10	0
Peach Topping, 1 ladle	21	0
Rainbow Sprinkles, 1 spoonful	13	0
Salsa, 1 ladle	2	0
Spice Drops, 1 spoonful	18	0
Strawberry Topping, 1 pump	23	0
Sunflower Seeds, 1 spoonful	2	<1
Whipped Topping, Nondairy, 1 spoonful	5	0

CONDIMENTS	C	F
Butter, 1 packet	0	0
Coffee Creamers, 1 packet	0	0
Croutons, 7 pieces	5	0
Honey, (1) packet	11	0
Jelly, (1) packet	9	0
Ketchup, 1 tablespoon	4	0

	C	F
Lemons, 1 slice	<1	0
Margarine, (1) packet	0	0
Margarine, melted, 1 ladle	<1	0
Mayonnaise, 1 tablespoon	0	0
Mustard, 1 tablespoon	1	<1
Nondairy Creamers, (1) packet	1	0
Peanut Butter, 1 tablespoon	3	0
Pickle Relish, sweet, 1 tablespoon	6	0
Red Pepper, crushed, 1 teaspoon	1	<1
Sour Cream, 1 spoonful	<1	0

DESSERTS	C	F
Ambrosia, 1 spoonful	23	1
Apple Crisp, 1 spoonful	31	2
Apple Pie - Reduced Sugar, 1 piece	24	2
Apple Strudel Bites, 1 piece	8	0
Banana Cream Pie - Reduced Sugar, 1 piece	21	<1
Banana Cream Pie, 1 piece	24	<1
Banana Nut Cake - Sugar Free, 1 piece	15	0
Banana Nut Cake, 1 piece	32	1
Bread Pudding, 1 spoonful	27	<1
Brownies, 1 brownie	24	<1
Carrot Cake, 1 piece	32	<1
Cheesecake, plain, 1 piece	29	0
Chocolate Cream Pie - Reduced Sugar, 1 piece	18	<1
Chocolate Decadence Cake, 1 piece	27	0
Cinnamon Sugared Donut Holes, 1 piece	5	0
Cobbler, Cherry, 1 spoonful	42	2
Cobbler, Peach, 1 spoonful	42	2
Cookie, Chocolate Chip, 1 cookie	18	<1
Cookie, Oatmeal Raisin, 1 cookie	15	1
Cookie, Peanut Butter, 1 cookie	16	<1
Cookie, Snickerdoodle, 1 cookie	18	0
Cookie, Sugar Free Chocolate-Chocolate Chip, 1 cookie	23	1
Cookie, Sugar Free Ranger, 1 cookie	11	<1
Devil's Food Cake, 1 piece	32	<1
Gelatin Whip, 1 spoonful	14	0

	C	F
Gelatin, Flavored, 1 spoonful	10	0
Glazed Donuts, 1 donut	16	0
Hot Fudge Sundae Cake, 1 spoonful	32	<1
Ice Cream Cone, 1 (cone only)	3	0
Pecan Pie, 1 piece	42	1
Pudding, Chocolate - Reduced Sugar, Reduced Calorie, 1 spoonful	14	0
Pudding, Chocolate, 1 spoonful	19	0
Pudding, Vanilla - Reduced Sugar, Reduced Calorie, 1 spoonful	14	0
Pudding, Vanilla, 1 spoonful	19	0
Pumpkin Pie, 1 piece	31	2
Raisin Fluff, 1 spoonful	25	<1
Reduced Sugar Pie - Cherry, 1 piece	16	0
Reduced Sugar Pie - Lemon, 1 piece	16	0
Reduced Sugar Pie - Lime, 1 piece	16	0
Reduced Sugar Pie - Orange, 1 piece	16	0
Reduced Sugar Pie - Raspberry, 1 piece	16	0
Reduced Sugar Pie - Strawberry, 1 piece	16	0
Rice Crispy Bars, 1 bar	16	0
Soft Serve Frozen Yogurt, Nonfat, NutraSweet, Vanilla, 4 fl oz	17	0
Soft Serve Frozen Yogurt, Nonfat, Strawberry, 4 fl oz	23	0
Soft Serve Frozen Yogurt, Nonfat, Vanilla, 4 fl oz	23	0
Soft Serve, Chocolate, 4 fl oz	24	<1
Soft Serve, Vanilla, 4 fl oz	25	<1
Strawberry Whip, 1 spoonful	17	0

IHOP®

	C	F
Pancakes: w/o Syrup or Butter, Buttermilk, 1 pancake	17	
Pancakes: w/o Syrup or Butter, Buttermilk short stack, 3 pancakes	51	
Pancakes: w/o Syrup or Butter, Buttermilk full stack, 5 pancakes	85	
Pancakes: w/o Syrup or Butter, Country Griddle Cakes, 1 pancake	19	
Pancakes: w/o Syrup or Butter, Harvest Grain 'N Nut, 1 pancake	20	
Pancakes: w/o Syrup or Butter, Crepe-Style, 2 oz	14	
Syrup: 1 tbsp	12	
Whipped Butter, 1 tbsp	0	
Waffles (Plain): regular, 1 waffle	37	
Waffles (Plain): Belgian, regular, 1 waffle	48	
Breakfast: Classic Combos: Cntry Fried Steak/Eggs, 1 serving	73	
Breakfast: Classic Combos: Fruity Country Griddle Cakes Combo, 1 serving	83	
Breakfast: Classic Combos: Harvest Grain 'N Nut Combo, 1 serving	80	
Breakfast: Classic Combos: T-Bone Steak & Eggs, 1 serving	63	
Signature, Rooty Tooty Fresh & Fruity, average, all flavors, 1 serving	84	
Omelette, Colorado Omelette: No pancakes, 1 serving	5	
Omelette, Colorado Omelette: with 3 buttermilk pancakes, 1 serving	66	
Omelette, The Big Steak Omelette: No pancakes, 1 serving	14	
Omlette, The Big Steak Omelette: with 3 buttermilk pancakes, 1 serving	75	
Burgers, Sourdough Bacon Burger Melt:burger only, 1 serving	37	
Burgers, Sourdough Bacon Burger Melt: with French Fries, 1 serving	104	
Burgers, Sourdough Bacon Burger Melt: with Onion Rings, 1 serving	64	
Burgers, Sourdough Bacon Burger Melt: with Salad & 2½ T. Reg Dressing, 1 serving	47	
Entrees: Old-Fashioned Pot Roast, 1 serving	30	
Entrees: Old-Fashioned Pot Roast with Mashed Potatoes, 1 serving	65	
Salad: Southwestern Chicken Fajita, with Tortilla Shell, 1 serving	48	

	C	F
Salad: Southwestern Chicken Fajita, w/o Tortilla Shell, 1 serving	35	

In-N-Out Burger®

	C	F
Burgers: Hamburger w. Onion, 1 serving	39	
Burgers: Hamburger w. Mustard/ Ketchup, no spread, 1 serving	41	
Burgers: Protein-Style, no bun, 1 serving	11	
Burgers: Cheeseburger w. Onion, 1 serving	39	
Burgers: Cheeseburger w. Mustard/ Ketchup, no spread, 1 serving	41	
Burgers: Cheeseburger Protein-Style, no bun, 1 serving	11	
Burgers: Double Double® (2 patty/ 2 sl. chse), 1 serving	39	
Burgers: Double Double® (2 patty/ 2 sl. chse) w. Mustard/Ketchup, no spread, 1 serving	41	
Burgers: Double Double® (2 patty/ 2 sl. chse) Protein-Style, no bun, 1 serving	11	
French Fries, 4.4 oz	54	
Drinks: Milk, 10 fl.oz	18	
Drinks: Coca-Cola, Dr Pepper, 16 fl.oz	54	
Drinks: Lemonade, 16 fl.oz	40	
Drinks: Root Beer, Seven-Up, 16 fl oz	54	
Shakes: average, all flavors, 15 fl.oz	83	

Jack in the Box®

	C	F
Breakfast Sausage, Egg & Cheese Biscuit, 1 each	33	2
Bacon, NA	0	0
Breakfast Jack®, NA	34	1
Extreme Sausage Sandwich, 1 each	35	2
French Toast Sticks, 4 pieces	57	2
Hash Brown, NA	13	2
Sausage Biscuit, 1 each	25	2
Sausage Croissant, 1 each	41	2
Sourdough Breakfast Sandwich, 1 each	36	2

	C	F
Supreme Croissant, 1 each	41	1
Ultimate Breakfast Sandwich, 1 each	52	1
Bacon Ultimate Cheeseburger, 1 each	42	1
Bacon Bacon Cheeseburger, 1 each	44	2
Double Cheeseburger, 1 each	32	1
Jack's Western Cheeseburger, 1 each	46	2
Jumbo Jack® with Cheese, 1 each	47	2
Jumbo Jack®, 1 each	45	2
Sourdough Jack®, 1 each	33	3
Ultimate Cheeseburger, 1 each	42	1
Hamburger, 1 each	30	2
Hamburger with Cheese, 1 each	31	2
Chicken Breast Pieces, 5 pieces	24	1
Chicken Fajita Pita, 1 each	35	3
Chicken Sandwich, 1 each	39	2
Chicken Supreme, 1 each	62	4
Chicken Teriyaki Bowl, 1 each	103	3
Fish & Chips, 1 serving	66	5
Grilled Chicken Fillet, 1 each	34	2
Jack's Spicy Chicken®, 1 each	53	3
Sourdough Grilled Chicken Club, 1 each	33	3
Taco, 1 each	16	2
Monster Taco, 1 each	22	3
Taco Sauce, 1 serving	0	0
Tartar Sauce, 1 serving	2	0
American Cheese, 1 slice	1	0
Barbeque Dipping Sauce, 1 serving	11	0
Buttermilk House Dipping Sauce, 1 serving	3	0
Frank's Red Hot Buffalo™ Dipping Sauce, 1 serving	2	0
Marinara Sauce, 1 serving	3	0
Mustard, 1 serving	1	0
Salsa, 1 serving	2	0
Sweet & Sour Dipping Sauce, 1 serving	11	0
Swiss-Style Cheese, 1 slice	1	0
Vinegar, 1 serving	0	0

	C	F
Country Crock™ Spread, 1 serving	0	0
Grape Jelly, 1 serving	9	0
Syrup, 1 serving	32	0
Ketchup, 1 serving	2	0
Sour Cream, 1 serving	2	0

Jamba Juice®

	C	F
Jamba Powerboost®, 1 each	103	7
Kiwi Berry Burner®, 1 each	112	5
Coldbuster®, 1 each	100	5
Protein Berry Pizazz, 1 each	102	6
Fruit Smoothies Banana Berry, 1 each	112	5
Fruit Smoothies Mango-A-Go-Go, 1 each	117	4
Fruit Smoothies Caribbean Passion®, 1 each	102	4
Fruit Smoothies Strawberries Wild®, 1 each	105	4
Fruit Smoothies Orange-A-Peel, 1 each	102	5
Fruit Smoothies Citrus Squeeze®, 1 each	93	5
Fruit Smoothies Orange Berry Blitz, 1 each	94	5
Fruit Smoothies Razzmatazz®, 1 each	112	4
Fruit Smoothies Berry Lime Sublime®, 1 each	104	6
Fruit Smoothies Peenya Kowlada®, 1 each	118	3
Fruit Smoothies Aloha Pineapple, 1 each	89	5
Fruit Smoothies Cranberry Craze®, 1 each	97	4
Fruit Smoothies Peach Pleasure®, 1 each	108	5
Fruit Smoothies Chocolate Moo'd®, 1 each	141	2
Fruit Smoothies Peanut Butter Moo'd, 1 each	139	5

Johnny Rockets®

	C	F
Hamburgers, #12, 1 serving	54	
Hamburgers, Chili Size, 1 serving	59	
Hamburgers, Original Burger, 1 serving	44	
Hamburgers, Patty Melt, 1 serving	51	
Hamburgers, Rocket Double, 1 serving	57	
Hamburgers, Rocket Single, 1 serving	56	
Hamburgers, Route 66, 1 serving	45	
Hamburgers, Smoke House, 1 serving	70	
Hamburgers, St. Louis, 1 serving	53	
Hamburgers, Streamliner, 1 serving	50	
Sandwiches, Chicken Club, 1 serving	62	
Sandwiches, Bacon, Lettuce & Tomato, 1 serving	44	
Sandwiches, Egg Salad, 1 serving	40	
Sandwiches, Grilled Breast of Chicken, 1 serving	54	
Sandwiches, Grilled Cheese, 1 serving	42	
Sandwiches, Grilled Ham & Cheese, 1 serving	48	
Sandwiches, Tuna Melt, 1 serving	42	
Sandwiches, Tuna Salad, 1 serving	41	
Others, Hot Dog, 1 serving	39	
Others, Chicken Club Salad w/ chicken tenders, 1 serving	37	
Others, Chicken Club Salad w/ Grilled Chicken Breast, 1 serving	8	
Others, Chicken Tenders, 1 serving	47	
Others, Chili Dog, 1 serving	46	
Others, Garden Salad, 1 serving	5	
Extras, Bacon, 0.7 oz	0	
Extras, Extra Patty, 3 oz	1	
Extras, Chili, 2.5 oz	3	
Extras, Grilled Onions or Mushrooms, 1 oz	2	
Starters, American Fries, 8 oz	77	
Starters, ½ Fries & ½ Rings, 9.3 oz	92	
Starters, Cheese Fries, 10 oz	77	

	C	F
Starters, Chili Bowl, 10 oz	12	
Starters, Chili Fries, 12 oz	76	
Starters, Onion Rings, 6.8 oz	22	
Desserts, Apple Pie, 1 serving	88	
Desserts, Hot Fudge Sundae, 1 serving	93	
Desserts, Hot Fudge Sundae A La Mode, 1 serving	26	
Drinks, Root beer, medium	43	
Drinks: Coke, Sprite, medium	43	
Drinks: Lemonade, medium	49	
Drinks: Float, medium	41	
Shakes: Chocolate, 20 fl oz	120	
Shakes: Strawberry, 20 fl oz	82	
Shakes: Vanilla, 20 fl oz	130	
Shakes: Extra for Malt,	10	

Kenny Rogers Roasters®

	C	F
Chicken, ½ Chicken, No Skin or Wing, 1 serving	1	
Chicken, ½ Chicken, with Skin, 1 serving	2	
Chicken, ¼ Dark Meat, No Skin, 1 serving	1	
Chicken, ¼ Dark Meat, with Skin, 1 serving	1	
Chicken, ¼ White Meat, No Skin or Wing, 1 serving	1	
Chicken, ¼ White Meat, with Skin, 1 serving	1	
Chicken, Grilled Breast Platter, 1 serving	100	
Chicken, Tenders, 3 tenders	24	
Chicken, Tenders Platter, 1 serving	119	
Chicken, Pies: Chicken Pot Pie, 1 serving	78	
Chicken, Pitas: BBQ Chicken, 1 serving	51	
Chicken, Chicken Caesar, 1 serving	34	
Chicken, Roasted Chicken, 1 serving	42	
Chicken, Turkey: Sliced Breast, 1 serving	0	

	C	F
Salads (No Dressing): Side Salad, 1 serving	5	
Salads (No Dressing): Chicken Caesar, 1 serving	18	
Salads (No Dressing): Pasta, 1 serving	28	
Salads (No Dressing): Roasted Chicken, 1 serving	19	
Salads (No Dressing): Sour Cream & Dill Pasta, 1 serving	20	
Salads (No Dressing): Tomato Cucumber, 1 serving	10	
Sandwiches, Chicken Tender, 1 serving	45	
Sandwiches, Chicken Tender Pita, 1 serving	45	
Sandwiches, Grilled Chicken, 1 serving	32	
Sandwiches, Turkey, 1 serving	30	
Side Dishes: Cinnamon Apples, 1 serving	41	
Side Dishes: Coleslaw, 1 serving	18	
Side Dishes: Cornbread Stuffing, 1 serving	34	
Side Dishes: Corn Cob, 1 serving	14	
Side Dishes: Corn Muffin, 1 serving	25	
Side Dishes: Sweet Corn Niblets, 1 serving	28	
Side Dishes: Creamy Parmesan Spinach	10	
Side Dishes: Honey Baked Beans, 1 serving	32	
Side Dishes: Italian Green Beans, 1 serving	10	
Side Dishes: Macaroni & Cheese, 1 serving	24	
Side Dishes: Potatoes, Baked Sweet, 1 serving	62	
Side Dishes: Garlic Parsley, 1 serving	37	
Side Dishes: Potato Salad, 1 serving	34	
Side Dishes: Real Mashed, 1 serving	39	
Side Dishes: Rice Pilaf, 1 serving	43	
Side Dishes: Steamed Vegetables, 1 serving	8	
Side Dishes: Zucchini & Squash Santa Fe, 1 serving	8	

	C	F
Soups: Chicken Noodle, 1 bowl	12	
Soups: Chicken Noodle, 1 cup	7	

KFC®

	C	F
BBQ Baked Beans, 1 serving	33	6
Biscuit, 1 each	20	<1
Chunky Chicken Pot Pie (after baking), 1 serving	69	5
Coleslaw, 1 serving	26	3
Colonel's Pies – Apple Pie Slice, 1 serving	44	0
Colonel's Pies – Pecan Pie Slice, 1 serving	66	2
Colonel's Pies – Strawberry Crème Pie Slice, 1 serving	32	2
Corn on the Cob, 1 serving	35	2
Crispy Caesar Twister, 1 serving	66	5
Double Chocolate Chip Cake, 1 serving	41	1
Extra Crispy Chicken - Breast or Thigh, average, 1 serving	15	<1
Extra Crispy Chicken - Drumstick, 1 serving	7	<1
Extra Crispy Chicken - Whole Wing, 1 serving	10	<1
Green Beans, 1 serving	7	3
Honey BBQ Crunch Melt, 1 serving	48	2
Honey BBQ Flavored Sandwich, 1 serving	37	2
Honey BBQ Pieces or Strips, 6 pieces	33	1
Hot & Spicy - Thigh, 1 serving	13	1
Hot & Spicy Chicken - Breast, 1 serving	23	1
Hot & Spicy Chicken - Whole Wing or Drumstick, 1 serving	9	<1
Hot Wings Pieces, 6 pieces	18	2
Little Bucket Parfait – Chocolate Cream, 1 serving	37	2
Little Bucket Parfait – Fudge Brownie, 1 serving	44	1
Little Bucket Parfait – Lemon Crème, 1 serving	62	4
Little Bucket Parfait – Strawberry Shortcake, 1 serving	33	1

	C	F
Macaroni & Cheese, 1 serving	21	2
Mashed Potatoes w/gravy, 1 serving	17	2
Mean Greens, 1 serving	11	5
Original Recipe Chicken - Darkmeat average, 1 serving	5	0
Original Recipe Chicken - White Meat, 1 serving	16	1
Original Recipe Sandwich w/ sauce, 1 serving	33	2
Original Recipe Sandwich w/o sauce, 1 serving	21	<1
Popcorn Chicken, small	21	0.2
Popcorn Chicken, large	36	0
Potato Salad, 1 serving	23	3
Potato Wedges, 1 serving	28	5
Strips, Crispy Colonel's, 3 pieces	18	1
Strips, Crispy Spicy, 3 pieces	23	<1
Tender Roast Sandwich w/ or w/o sauce average, 1 serving	25	1
Triple Crunch Sandwich w/sauce, 1 serving	39	2
Triple Crunch Sandwich w/o sauce, 1 serving	29	2
Triple Crunch Zinger Sand. w/ sauce, 1 serving	39	2
Triple Crunch Zinger Sand. w/o sauce, 1 serving	36	2
Twister Wrap, 1 serving	52	4

Kohr Bros ®

	C	F
Frozen Custard, Chocolate flavored, ½ cup	18	
Frozen Custard, Orange Sherbert flavored, ½ cup	21	
Frozen Custard, Vanilla flavored, ½ cup	16	

Krispy Kreme Doughnuts®

	C	F
Glazed Mini Cruller, 3 each	32	1
Chocolate Enrobed Doughnut Holes, 3 each	27	2
Honey Bun, 1 each	44	1

	C	F
Coconut Crème Pie, 1 each	61	2
Peach Pie, 1 each	51	0
Cherry Pie, 1 each	56	1
Apple Pie, 1 each	54	3
Glazed Doughnut (Ring), 1 each	23	2
Chocolate Iced Glazed Ring w/Sprinkles, 1 each	36	>1
Chocolate Iced Glazed (Ring), 1 each	36	1
Maple Iced Glazed (Ring), 1 each	34	>1
Cinnamon Bun, 1 each	28	>1
Sugar Doughnut, 1 each	21	0
Cinnamon Twist, 1 each	33	1
Glazed Twist, 1 each	28	>1
Traditional, 1 each	25	>1
Traditional Chocolate Iced, 1 each	36	>1
Powdered Sugar, 1 each	33	>1
Glazed Cruller, 1 each	26	>1
Chocolate Iced Glazed Cruller, 1 each	35	>1
Devil's Food Old-Fashioned, 1 each	41	5
Glazed Blueberry Old-Fashioned, 1 each	37	1
Old-Fashioned Sour Cream, 1 each	41	0
Vanilla Iced with Sprinkles, 1 each	39	>1
Plain Mini Cake, 4 each	27	1
Powdered Sugar Mini Cake, 3 each	26	>1
Chocolate (Enrobed) Mini Cake, 3 each	26	3
Old Fashioned Honey & Oat, 1 each	36	>2
Apple Filled Cinnamon Sugar Coated, 1 each	35	3
Blueberry Filled Powdered Sugar Coated, 1 each	33	1
Chocolate Iced Cream Filled, 1 each	39	4
Chocolate Iced Custard Filled, 1 each	39	5
Glazed Cherry Filled, 1 each	36	5
Glazed Crème Filled, 1 each	39	1
Glazed Raspberry Filled, 1 each	36	2
Powdered Raspberry Filled, 1 each	36	>1
Vanilla Iced Crème Filled, 1 each	41	5
Vanilla Iced Custard Filled, 1 each	33	>1

	C	F
Glazed Lemon Filled, 1 each	34	>1
Glazed Custard Filled, 1 each	34	>1
Powdered Strawberry Filled, 1 each	26	>1
Powdered Sugar Doughnut Holes, 3 each	23	2
Glazed Doughnut Holes, 3 each	25	1

Leeann Chin®

ENTREES

	C	F
Beef and Vegetable Seasonal Stir Fry, 6 oz	24	2
Cashew Chicken, 6 oz	21	3
Chicken and Vegetable Seasonal Stir Fry, 6 oz	22	2
Lemon Chicken, 6 oz	32	0
Orange Chicken, 6 oz	44	2
Peking Chicken, 6 oz	31	0
Pork and Vegetable Seasonal Stir Fry, 6 oz	23	2
Sesame Chicken, 6 oz	42	1
Shrimp and Vegetable Rotating Stir Fry, 6 oz	22	2
Sweet and Sour Chicken, 6 oz	47	2
Vegetable Rotating Stir Fry, 6 oz	24	2

RICE, LO MEIN, & NOODLES

	C	F
Asian Noodles, 4 oz	33	2
Beef Lo Mein, 6 oz	27	0
Vegetable Fried Rice, 4 oz	36	1
White Rice, 4 oz	38	0
Young Jewel Rice, 4 oz	37	1

SALADS / OTHER

	C	F
Cantonese Noodle Salad, 1 salad	38	3
Chinese Chicken Salad, (1)	23	2
Cream Cheese Puffs, 1 cheese puff	10	0
Egg Rolls, 1 roll	20	2
Oyster Wings, 1 wing	5	0
Potstickers, 1 potsticker	6	1

Little Caesar®

	C	F
Pizzas, 12" Round: Cheese or Pepperoni, ⅛ pizza, 1 slice	23	
Pizzas, 12" Thin Crust: Cheese or Pepperoni, ⅛ pizza, 1 slice	13	
Pizzas, 14" Round: Cheese, Meatsa or Pepperoni, average, 1/10 pizza, 1 slice	25	
Pizzas, 14" Round: Supreme or Veggie, average, 1/10 pizza, 1 slice	32	
Pizzas, 14" Thin Crust: Cheese or Pepperoni, 1/10 pizza, 1 slice	14	
Pizzas, 16" Round Cheese or Pepperoni, 1/12 pizza, 1 slice	27	
Pizzas, 18" Round: Cheese or Pepperoni, 1/14 pizza, 1 slice	30	
Pizzas, Large Deep Dish: Cheese or Pepperoni, average, ⅛ pizza, 1 slice	38	
Pizzas, medium Deep Dish: Cheese, ⅛ pizza, 1 slice	27	
Extras, Baby Pan! Pan!, 1 piece, 5.0 oz	34	
Extras, Chicken Wings (1), 1 wing	0	
Extras, Crazy Bread: 1 stick, 1 stick	15	
Extras, Cinnamon, 2 sticks, 2 sticks	19	
Extras, Crazy Sauce, 4 oz	9	
Extras, Italian Cheese Bread, 1 piece	13	
Sandwiches, Deli: Ham & Cheese, 1 sandwich	66	
Sandwiches, Italian, 1 sandwich	66	
Sandwiches, Veggie, 1 sandwich	67	
Side Salads: Antipasto, 1 serving	6	
Side Salads: Caesar, 1 serving	12	
Side Salads: Greek, 1 serving	11	
Side Salads: Tossed, 1 serving	15	
Salad Dressings: Caesar, 1 serving	1	
Salad Dressings: Greek, 1 serving	0	
Salad Dressings: Italian, 1 serving	2	
Salad Dressings: Ranch, 1 serving	2	
Salad Dressings: Fat Free: Italian, 1 serving	5	

Long John Silver's®

	C	F
Sandwich, Ultimate Fish, 1 serving	48	
Sandwich, Fish, 1 serving	41	
Sandwich, Chicken , 1 serving	41	
Sides: Fries, regular	34	
Sides: Fries, large, 5 oz	56	
Sides: Cheese Sticks (3), 3 sticks	12	
Sides: Coleslaw, 4 oz	15	
Sides: Corn Cobbette, no butter, 1 serving	14	
Sides: Crumblies, 1 oz	14	
Sides: Hush puppy(I), 1 hush puppy	9	
Sides: Rice, 4 oz	34	
Soup: Clam Chowder, 1 bowl	23	
Chicken: Battered Plank, 1 piece	9	
Seafood: Battered Fish, 1 piece	16	
Seafood: Battered Shrimp, 1 piece	3	
Seafood: Breaded Clams, 1 order	22	
Desserts: Chocolate Cream Pie, 1 serving	24	
Desserts: Pecan Pie, 1 serving	55	
Desserts: Pineapple Cream Pie, 1 serving	39	

Maggie Moo's ®

Fat Free Ice Cream, ½ cup	18	0
Low-Carb NSA (No Sugar Added) Ice Cream, ½ cup	11	0
Sorbet, ½ cup	22	0
Udderly Cream, ½ cup	18	0

McDonald's®

Cheddar Bacon Sausage McMuffin, 1 each	27	
Egg McMuffin, 1 each	27	
Sausage McMuffin, 1 each	26	
Sausage McMuffin with Egg, 1 each	27	
English Muffin, 1 each	25	
Sausage Biscuit, 1 each	30	
Sausage Biscuit with Egg, 1 each	31	

	C	F
Bacon, Egg & Cheese Biscuit, 1 each	31	
Biscuit, 1 each	30	
Ham and Egg Cheese Bagel, 1 each	58	
Spanish Omelet Bagel, 1 each	60	
Steak and Egg Cheese Bagel, 1 each	57	
Sausage, 1 each	0	
Scrambled Eggs (2), 1 serving	1	
Hash Browns, 1 each	14	
Hotcakes (plain), 1 serving	58	
Hotcakes (margarine, 2 pats, & syrup), 1 serving	104	
Breakfast Burrito, 1 each	24	
Low fat Apple Bran Muffin, 1 each	61	
Apple Danish, 1 each	47	
Cheese Danish, 1 each	45	
Cinnamon Roll, 1 each	50	
Chicken Breast Parmesan, 1 each	47	
Hamburger, 1 each	35	
Cheeseburger, 1 each	36	
Quarter Pounder®, 1 each	37	
Quarter Pounder® with Cheese, 1 each	38	
Nuts (on Sundaes), 1 serving	2	
Butterfinger® McFlurry™, 1 each	90	
M&M® McFlurry™, 1 each	90	
Oreo® McFlurry™, 1 each	82	
Baked Apple Pie, 1 each	34	
Chocolate Chip Cookies, 1 pkg.	37	
McDonaldland Cookies, 1 pkg.	38	
Vanilla Shake, small, 1 each	59	
Chocolate Shake, small, 1 each	60	
Strawberry Shake, small, 1 each	60	
Big Mac®, 1 each	47	
Big N' Tasty®, 1 each	39	
Big N' Tasty® with Cheese, 1 each	40	
Crispy Chicken, 1 each	54	
Filet-O-Fish®, 1 each	45	
Chicken McGrill®, 1 each	46	
Chicken McGrill® (plain w/o mayo), 1 each	45	

	C	F
French Fries, small, 1 serving	26	
French Fries, medium, 1 serving	57	
French Fries, large, 1 serving	68	
French Fries, super size, 1 serving	77	
Chicken McNuggets®, 4 pieces	13	
Chicken McNuggets®, 6 pieces	20	
Chicken McNuggets®, 9 pieces	29	
Hot Mustard Sauce, 1 pkg	7	
Barbeque Sauce, 1 pkg	10	
Sweet 'N Sour Sauce, 1 pkg	11	
Honey, 1 pkg	12	
Honey Mustard, 1 pkg	3	
Light Mayonnaise, 1 pkg	1	
Chef Salad, 1 serving	5	
Garden Salad, 1 serving	4	
Grilled Chicken Caesar Salad, 1 serving	3	
Croutons, 1 pkg	9	
Caesar Dressing, 1 pkg	5	
Fat Free Herb Vinaigrette Dressing, 1 pkg	8	
Honey Mustard Dressing, 1 pkg	13	
Ranch Dressing, 1 pkg	3	
Red French Reduced Calorie Dressing, 1 pkg	18	
1000 Island Dressing, 1 pkg.	11	
Fruit 'N Yogurt Parfait, 1 each	76	
Fruit 'N Yogurt Parfait w/o Granola, 1 each	53	
Vanilla Reduced Fat Ice Cream Cone, 1 each	23	
Strawberry Sundae, 1 each	50	
Hot Caramel Sundae, 1 each	61	
Hot Fudge Sundae, 1 each	52	

Mrs. Fields Cookies®

	C	F
Brownie, Butterscotch Blondie, 1 brownie	29	
Brownie, Double Fudge, 1 brownie	32	
Brownie, Mint Fudge, 1 brownie	35	
Brownie, Pecan Fudge, 1 brownie	31	

	C	F
Brownie, Pecan Pie, 1 brownie	8	
Brownie, Pecan Pie Chocolate Chip, 1 brownie	24	
Brownie, special Walnut Fudge & Blondie, 1 brownie	35	
Brownie, Toffee Fudge, 1 brownie	35	
Brownie, Walnut Fudge, 1 brownie	31	
Cakes, Blueberry, 3 oz	36	
Cakes, Carrot Cake, 3 oz	37	
Cakes, Chocolate, 3 oz	35	
Cakes, Chocolate Chip, 3 oz	45	
Cakes, Cinnamon Sugar Pecan, slice, 2.1 oz	32	
Cakes, Lemon Bundt, slice, 2.1 oz	40	
Cakes, Raspberry, 3 oz	36	
Cakes, Raspberry Chocolate Chip, 2.1 oz	36	
Cookies, Bite Size Nibblers: Cinn. Sugar (2), 2 cookies	17	
Cookies, Bite Size Nibblers: Debra's Special (2), 2 cookies	13	
Cookies, Bite Size Nibblers: Peanut Butter (2), 2 cookies	13	
Cookies, Bite Size Nibblers: Semi-Sweet Chocolate (2), 2 cookies	15	
Cookies, Bite Size Nibblers: Triple Chocolate (2), 2 cookies	15	
Cookies, Bite Size Nibblers: White Chunk Macadamia (2), 2 cookies	13	
Cookies, Cinnamon Sugar (1), 1 cookie	41	
Cookies, Coconuts Macadamia (1), 1 cookie	39	
Cookies, Debra's Special (1), 1 cookie	39	
Cookies, Milk Chocolates Walnuts (1), 1 cookie	37	
Cookies, Milk Chocolate Macadamia (1), 1 cookie	36	
Cookies, Milk Chocolate, no nuts (1), 1 cookie	38	
Cookies, Oatmeal Chocolate Chip (1), 1 cookie	40	
Cookies, Oatmeal Raisin (1), 1 cookie	29	

	C	F
Cookies, Peanut Butter (1), 1 cookie	34	
Cookies, Semi-Sweet Chocolate (1), 1 cookie	40	
Cookies, Semi-Sweet Chocolate w. Walnuts (1), 1 cookie	38	
Cookies, Triple Chocolate (1), 1 cookie	31	
Cookies, White Chunk Macadamia (1), 1 cookie	37	

Nathan's Famous®

	C	F
Burger, ¼ lb, 1 serving	42	
Burger, ¼ lb w/ cheese, 1 serving	45	
Burger, Bacon Cheeseburger, 1 serving	43	
Burger, Super Bacon Cheeseburger, 1 serving	42	
Cheesesteaks: Chicken, 1 serving	62	
Cheesesteaks: Original, 1 serving	50	
Cheesesteaks: Supreme, 1 serving	61	
Fish Sandwich, 1 serving	41	
Hot Dogs: Nathan's Famous, 1 Hot Dog	22	
Sides: French Fries: regular	46	
Sides: French Fries: large	65	
Sides: French Fries: super	101	
Nuggets (6), 3.5 oz	20	
Onion Rings, 5.6 oz	36	

Noah's Bagels®

	C	F
Asiago Cheese Topped Bagel, (1)	78	2
Blueberry Bagel, (1)	79	3
Blueberry Bagel, Shtick, (1)	94	3
Chocolate Chip Bagel, (1)	80	3
Chopped Garlic Bagel, (1)	78	2
Cinnamon Raisin Bagel, (1)	80	2
Cinnamon Sugar Bagel, (1)	74	2
Cinnamon Sugar Bagel, Shtick, (1)	79	2
Cracked Pepper Bagel, (1)	78	3
Cranberry Orange Bagel, (1)	80	3

	C	F
Egg Bagel, (1)	76	2
Everything Bagel, (1)	77	2
New York Rye Bagel, (1)	76	3
Onion Bagel, (1)	77	3
Onion with Asiago Bagel, Shtick, (1)	71	2
Plain Bagel, (1)	77	2
Poppyseed Bagel, (1)	78	2
Pumpernickel Bagel, (1)	76	3
Salt Bagel, (1)	77	2
Sesame Seed Bagel, (1)	77	2
Sun-Dried Tomato Bagel, (1)	77	3
Whole Wheat Bagel, (1)	73	4
Whole Wheat Bagel, (1) w/ Sesame & Sunflower Seeds	74	4
Cream Cheese (Raskis), Garden Vegetable Spread, 2 tbl	2	0

Noodles & Company®

	C
Classics: Buttered Noodles S Parm., 1 serving	134
Classics: Chicken Noodle Soup, 1 serving	37
Classics: Mushroom Stroganoff, 1 serving	116
Classics: Pad Thai, 1 serving	147
Classics: Pesto Cavatappi, 1 serving	89
Classics: Tomato Marinara, 1 serving	87
Classics: Wisconsin Mac & Cheese, 1 serving	99
Noodle-Less: Chicken Rustica, 1 serving	11
Noodle-Less: Mediterranean Mixed Grill, 1 serving	12
Noodle-Less: Shrimp Curry Saute, 1 serving	20
Noodle-Less: Sweet Chili Chicken, 1 serving	29
Specialties: Bangkok Curry, 1 serving	71
Specialties: Indonesian Peanut Saute, 1 serving	128
Specialties: Japanese Pan Noodle, 1 serving	128
Specialties: Pasta Fresca, 1 serving	93

	C	F
Specialties: PenneRosa, 1 serving	70	
Specialties: Thai Curry Soup, 1 serving	49	
Specialties: Whole Grain Tuscan Fettuccine, 1 serving	70	
Salads: Caesar Salad, 1 serving	28	
Salads: Chinese Chop Salad, 1 serving	33	
Salads: Market Salad w. Fat Free Dressing, 1 serving	43	
Salads: Mediterranean Salad, 1 serving	11	
Salads: Spicy Peanut Noodle Salad, 1 serving	83	
Salads: Spicy Thai Caesar Salad, 1 serving	11	
Sides: Potstickers (3), 3 pieces	55	
Sides: Cucumber Tomato Salad, 1 serving	21	
Sides: Grilled Chicken Breast, 1 serving	0	
Sides: Sauteed Organic Tofu, 1 serving	3	
Sides: Sauteed Shrimp, 8 pieces	1	
Sides: Thin-Cut Grilled Steak, 4 oz	1	
Sides: Veggie Trio, 5 oz	7	

Old Country Buffet®

	C	F
Entrees: BBQ Beef Ribs, 5 oz	7	
Entrees: BBQ Smoked Sausage, 2.8 oz	9	
Entrees: Beef Patties w. Mushroom Gravy, 1 serving	2	
Entrees: Carved: Beef Brisket, 3 oz	1	
Entrees: Ham, 3 oz	0	
Entrees: Peppered Pork Loin, 3 oz	0	
Entrees: Roast Beef, 3 oz	0	
Entrees: Roast Turkey, 3 oz	0	
Entrees: Salmon Filet, 3 oz	0	
Entrees: Cheese Enchiladas, 4.1 oz	13	
Entrees: Chicken Wings: Hot, Crummies, 1	0	
Entrees: Chicken Wings: Hot, 1	0	

	C	F
Entrees: Teriyaki, Drummie, 0.9 oz	2	
Entrees: Teriyaki, Wing, 0.45 oz	2	
Entrees: Chicken Hand-Breaded Fried: Breast, 5 oz	3	
Entrees: Chicken Hand-Breaded Fried: Drumstick, 1.4 oz	0	
Entrees: Chicken Hand-Breaded Fried: Thigh, 3.1 oz	4	
Entrees: Chicken, Traditional Baked: Breast, 1 piece	0	
Entrees: Chicken, Traditional Baked: Drumstick, 1.4 oz	0	
Entrees: Chicken, Traditional Baked: Thigh, 3.2 oz	0	
Entrees: Fish: Patties: Broiled, 2.5 oz	13	
Entrees: Fish: Patties: Baked, 3 oz	0	
Entrees: Fish: Patties: Fried, 1.3 oz	9	
Entrees: Meatloaf, 3, 2 oz	9	
Entrees: Shrimp, fried, 6 shrimp	11	
Entrees: Smoked Sausage & Sauerkraut, 1 serving	3	
Entrees: Spanish Rice, 3 oz	9	
Salads: California Coleslaw, 3.5 oz	22	
Salads: Macaroni Vegetable Salad, 3.5 oz	20	
Salads: Marinated Vegetables, 3.5 oz	6	
Salads: Seven Layer Salad, 2.6 oz	4	
Salads: Tossed Green Salad, 1 cup	1	
Sides: Potato: Baked, 6.3 oz	39	
Sides: Potato: Mashed, 5 oz	30	
Soups; Chili Bean, 4 fl oz	9	
Soups; Corn Chowder, 4 fl oz	15	
Soups; Navy Bean w. Ham, 4 fl oz	10	
Desserts: Cheesecake, plain, 1 piece	29	
Desserts: Chocolate Decadence, 1 piece	27	
Desserts: Cookie, Sugar Free Ranger, 1 cookie	11	
Desserts: Hot Fudge Sundae, 1 serving	32	
Desserts: Pumpkin Pie, reduced sugar, 1 slice	31	
Desserts: Pudding: Chocolate, 1 spoon, 3 oz	19	

	C	F
Desserts: Pudding: Chocolate, Reduced Sugar/Calorie, 3 oz	14	
Desserts: Pudding: Vanilla, 1 spoon, 3 oz	19	
Desserts: Soft Serve Ice Cream, average, 4 oz	24	

The Old Spaghetti Factory®

	C	F
Lunch Entrees: Fettuccine Alfredo, 1 serving	71	
Lunch Entrees: PotPourri, 10 oz	137	
Starter, Garlic Cheese Bread, 13.5 oz	105	
Lunch Entrees: Lasagna, 16 oz	36	
Lunch Entrees: Chicken Marsala, 18 oz	55	
Lunch Entrees: Chicken Parmigiana, 19 oz	84	
Lunch Entrees: Spinach & Cheese Ravioli, 12 oz	59	
Lunch Entrees: Spinach Tortellini w. Alfredo, 12 oz	82	
Lunch Entrees: Spaghetti: w. Clam Sauce, 10 oz	56	
Lunch Entrees: Spaghetti: w. Meat Sauce, 10 oz	55	
Lunch Entrees: Spaghetti: w. Meatballs, 13.5 oz	62	
Lunch Entrees: Spaghetti: w. Meat Sauce & Marinara, 9.2 oz	53	
Lunch Entrees: Spaghetti: w. Marinara / Mushroom / Tomato Sauce, 13.7 oz	52	
Lunch Entrees: Spaghetti: w. Sausage & Meat Sauce, 13.7 oz	57	
Lunch Entrees: Spaghetti: w. Tomato & Meat Sauce, 10 oz	56	

Orange Julius®

	C	F
Original (Orange, Strawberry): small, average, 16 fl oz	55	
Original (Orange, Strawberry): medium, average, 20 fl oz	68	
Original (Orange, Strawberry): large, average, 32 fl oz	109	

	C	F
Classic Smoothy Drinks: Bananarilla; Tropical, average, 16 fl oz	56	
Classic Smoothy Drinks: Cool Cappuccino, average, 16 fl oz	69	
Classic Smoothy Drinks: Pina Colada; Tripleberry, average, 16 fl oz	70	
Classic Smoothy Drinks: Strawberry Banana, 16 fl oz	77	
20 fl.oz size ~ Add 25% to above figures,		
32 fl.oz size ~ Double the above figures,		
Premium: Berry Lively, Blackberry Toner, 20 fl oz	100	
Premium: Blackberry Storm, 20 fl oz	130	
Premium: Blueberrathon, 20 fl oz	90	
Premium: Chai Tea Dragon, 20 fl oz	110	
Premium: Cocoa Latte Swirl, 20 fl oz	122	
Premium: Fruitasia, 20 fl oz	90	
Premium: Orange Swirl, 20 fl oz	96	
Premium: Raspberry Crush, 20 fl oz	83	
Premium: Strawb. Treasure, Raspb. Creme, 20 fl oz	103	
Premium: Strawberry Xtreme, 20 fl oz	87	
Premium: Tart'N'Berry, 20 fl oz	102	
Premium: Tropi-Colada, 20 fl oz	110	
Add Ins: Banana, medium	27	
Add Ins: Nutrifiers average, all types, ¼ oz	4	

Outback Steakhouse®

	C	F
Aussie-tizers, Aussie Cheese Fries, 28 oz	240	
Aussie-tizers, Bloomin' Onion w/ dressing, 1 serving	241	
Aussie-tizers, Bloomin' Onion w/ dressing, ¼ serving	60	
Aussie-tizers, Gold Coast Coconut Shrimp, 1 serving	97	
Aussie-tizers, Grilled Shrimp on the Barbie, 1 serving	32	

	C	F
Aussie-tizers, Kookaburra Wings w/ sauce, 10 wings	65	
Aussie-tizers, Lobster Crab Cakes, 2 cakes	33	
Steaks: Meat Only: Michael J. "Crocodile" Dundee: New York Strip, 14 oz	0	
Steaks: Meat Only: Outback Special, Sirloin, 12 oz	0	
Steaks: Meat Only: Prime Minister's Prime Ribs: 8 oz cut	0	
Steaks: Meat Only: Prime Minister's Prime Ribs: 12 oz cut	0	
Steaks: Meat Only: Prime Minister's Prime Ribs: 16 oz cut	0	
Rockhampton Rib-Eye au jus, 14 oz	0	
The Melbourne, Porterhouse, 20 oz	0	
The Melbourne, Porterhouse, Lean meat only, 1 serving	0	
Victoria's Filet, Tenderloin, 9 oz	0	
Sides: Aussie Chips w Ketchup, 1 serving	100	
Sides: Fresh Veggies, 1 serving	14	
Sides: Grilled Onions, 7.5 oz	19	
Sides: Jacket Potato, plain, 1 serving	63	
Sides: Jacket Potato, w. Butter/ Cheese, 1 serving	63	
Sides: Mushrooms, Sauteed, 1 serving	12	
Desserts: Cheesecake Olivia, 1 serving	79	
Desserts: Choc. Thunder from Down Under, 1 serving	134	

Panda Express®

	C	F
Black Pepper Chicken, 5 oz	11	1
Orange Chicken, 5 oz	31	0
Chicken with Mushrooms, 5 oz	9	1
Chicken with String Beans, 5 oz	12	2
Spicy Chicken with Peanuts, 5 oz	28	5
Beef & Broccoli, 5 oz	13	2
Sweet and Sour Pork, 4 oz	8	0
Sweet & Sour Sauce, 2 oz	16	0

	C	F
Mixed Vegetables, 5 oz	11	2
Hot & Sour Soup, 12 oz	13	0
Egg Flower Soup, 12 oz	18	1
Vegetable Fried Rice, 8 oz	47	1
Steamed Rice, 8 oz	48	1
Lo Mein, 8 oz	37	2
Vegetable Chow Mein, 8 oz	43	3
Egg Rolls, 2 pieces	30	1

Papa John's®

	C	F
Original Crust (14"): ⅛ whole: All the Meats w. Beef, 1 slice	17	
Original Crust (14"): ⅛ whole: BBQ Chicken & Bacon, 1 slice	11	
Original Crust (14"): ⅛ whole: Cheese, 1 slice	12	
Original Crust (14"): ⅛ whole: Garden Fresh, 1 slice	9	
Original Crust (14"): ⅛ whole: Hawaiian BBQ Chicken, 1 slice	11	
Original Crust (14"): ⅛ whole: Pepperoni, 1 slice	13	
Original Crust (14"): ⅛ whole: Sausage, 1 slice	15	
Original Crust (14"): ⅛ whole: Spinach Alfredo/Chicken, 1 slice	11	
Original Crust (14"): ⅛ whole: The Works, 1 slice	11	
Thin Crust (14"): ⅛ whole: All the Meats: w. Beef, 1 slice	20	
Thin Crust (14"): ⅛ whole: BBQ Chicken & Bacon, 1 slice	14	
Thin Crust (14"): ⅛ whole: Cheese, 1 slice	14	
Thin Crust (14"): ⅛ whole: Garden Fresh, 1 slice	12	
Thin Crust (14"): ⅛ whole: Grilled Chicken Alfredo, 1 slice	13	
Thin Crust (14"): ⅛ whole: Grilled Chicken Club, 1 slice	14	
Thin Crust (14"): ⅛ whole: Hawaiian BBQ Chicken, 1 slice	14	
Thin Crust (14"): ⅛ whole: Pepperoni, 1 slice	15	

	C	F
Thin Crust (14"): ⅛ whole: Sausage, 1 slice	18	
Thin Crust (14"): ⅛ whole: Spicy Italian, 1 slice	14	
Thin Crust (14"): ⅛ whole: Spinach Alfredo/Chicken, 1 slice	14	
Thin Crust (14"): ⅛ whole: The Works, 1 slice	14	
Side Orders: Bread Sticks, 1 stick	2	
Side Orders: Cheese Sticks, 2 sticks	16	
Side Orders: Papa's Chickenstrips, 2 strips	8	
Side Orders: Papa's Cinnapie, 2 slices, 2 oz	8	
Sauce: Garlic, 1 oz, 1 oz	17	
Sauce: Honey Mustard, 1 oz	15	
Sauce: Pizza, 1 oz	0	

Perkin's® Family Restaurant

	C	F
Entrees: Chicken Dinner, 1 serving	60	
Entrees: Fish Dinner, 1 serving	60	
Entrees: Fruit Cup, 1 serving	12	
Entrees: Lite & Healthy, 1 serving	15	
Omelette: Country Club, 1 serving	6	
Omelette: Deli Ham & Cheese, 1 serving	8	
Omelette: Everything Omelette, 1 serving	9	
Omelette: Granny's Country Omelette, 1 serving	7	
Omelette: Granny's Country Omelette Hash Browns, 1 serving	57	
Salads: Chef's, Mini, 1 salad	7	
Muffins: Banana, 1 muffin	78	
Muffins: Blueberry, Pumpkin, 1 muffin	78	
Muffins: Bran, 1 muffin	94	
Muffins: Carrot, 1 muffin	55	
Muffins: Chocolate Chips, 1 muffin	81	
Muffins: Cranberry Nut, 1 muffin	75	
Muffins: Lemon Poppyseed, 1 muffin	88	
Muffins: Oat Bran, 1 muffin	68	

	C	F
Muffins: Peaches & Cream; Apple, average, 1 muffin	72	
Muffins: Raspberry & Cream, 1 muffin	81	
Pancakes: Buttermilk (1), no syrup, 1 pancake	20	
Pancakes: Short Stack (3), no syrup, 3 pancakes	60	
Pancakes: Regular Stack (5), no syrup, 5 pancakes	100	
Pies: Apple Pie, ⅙ pie, 1 slice	56	
Pies: Wildberry, ⅙ pie, 1 slice	66	
Cake: Bundt, w. Icing (sugar free), 1 piece	70	

P F Chang's®

APPETIZERS

	C	F
Appetizers: Crab Wonton w/ Plum Sauce, 1 serving	51	
Appetizers: Harvest Spring Rolls, 1 serving	106	
Appetizers: Lettuce Wraps: Soothing Chicken, 1 serving	92	
Appetizers: Lettuce Wraps: Vegetarian, 1 serving	71	
Appetizers: Peking Dumplings: Pan-Fried, 1 serving	31	
Appetizers: Peking Dumplings: Steamed, 1 serving	31	
Appetizers: Seared Ahi Tuna w. Mustard, 1 serving	18	
Appetizers: Shanghai Street Dumplings, 1 serving	90	
Appetizers: Shrimp Dumplings: Pan-Fried, 1 serving	20	
Appetizers: Shrimp Dumplings: Steamed w. Ginger Sauce, 1 serving	26	
Appetizers: Spare Ribs: Northern Style, 1 serving	6	
Appetizers: Spare Ribs: w. Barbecue Sauce, 1 serving	47	
Appetizers: Vegetable Dumplings: Pan-Fried, 1 serving	47	
Appetizers: Vegetable Dumplings: Steamed, 1 serving	47	

MAIN DISHES,	C	F
Beef: A La Mongolian, 1 serving	18	
Beef: A La Orange Peel, 1 serving	69	
Beef: A La Sichuan, 1 serving	55	

DESSERTS

	C	F
Desserts: New York Style Cheesecake, 1 serving	72	

Pizza Hut®

	C	F
The Sicilian Pizza Cheese, 1 slice	31	2
The Sicilian Pizza Beef Topping, 1 slice	31	2
The Sicilian Pizza Ham, 1 slice	30	2.6
The Sicilian Pizza Pepperoni, 1 slice	31	2
The Sicilian Pizza Italian Sausage, 1 slice	31	2.8
The Sicilian Pizza Pork Topping, 1 slice	31	2
The Sicilian Pizza Meat Lover's®, 1 slice	31	2
The Sicilian Pizza Veggie Lover's®, 1 slice	32	2
The Sicilian Pizza Pepperoni Lover's®, 1 slice	31	2
The Sicilian Pizza Supreme, 1 slice	32	2
The Sicilian Pizza Super Supreme, 1 slice	32	2
The Sicilian Pizza Chicken Supreme, 1 slice	32	2
Stuffed Crust Cheese—Large, 1 slice	39	3
Stuffed Crust Beef—Large, 1 slice	40	3
Stuffed Crust Ham—Large, 1 slice	39	3
Stuffed Crust Pepperoni—Large, 1 slice	39	3
Stuffed Crust Ital. Sausage—Large, 1 slice	40	3
Stuffed Crust Meat Lover's®—Large, 1 slice	40	3
Stuffed Crust Pork—Large, 1 slice	40	3
Stuffed Crust Veggie Lover's®—Large, 1 slice	42	3
Stuffed Crust Pepperoni Lover's®—Large, 1 slice	40	3
Stuffed Crust Supreme—Large, 1 slice	41	3

	C	F
Stuffed Crust Super Supreme–Large, 1 slice	41	3
Stuffed Crust Chicken Supreme–Large, 1 slice	41	3
Hand-Tossed Pizza–Medium-Sized Cheese, 1 slice	28	2
Hand-Tossed Pizza–Medium-Sized Beef Topping, 1 slice	29	3
Hand-Tossed Pizza–Medium-Sized Ham, 1 slice	28	2
Hand-Tossed Pizza–Medium-Sized Pepperoni, 1 slice	28	2
Hand-Tossed Pizza–Medium-Sized Italian Sausage, 1 slice	28	2
Hand-Tossed Pizza–Medium-Sized Pork Topping, 1 slice	29	3
Hand-Tossed Pizza–Medium-Sized Meat Lover's®, 1 slice	28	2
Hand-Tossed Pizza–Medium-Sized Veggie Lover's®, 1 slice	29	2
Hand-Tossed Pizza–Medium-Sized Pepperoni Lover's®, 1 slice	27	2
Hand-Tossed Pizza–Medium-Sized Supreme, 1 slice	29	3
Hand-Tossed Pizza–Medium-Sized Super Supreme, 1 slice	29	2
Hand-Tossed Pizza–Medium-Sized Chicken Supreme, 1 slice	29	2
Thin 'n Crispy Pizza–Medium-Sized Cheese, 1 slice	22	2
Thin 'n Crispy Pizza–Medium-Sized Beef Topping, 1 slice	22	2
Thin 'n Crispy Pizza–Medium-Sized Ham, 1 slice	21	2
Thin 'n Crispy Pizza–Medium-Sized Pepperoni, 1 slice	21	2
Thin 'n Crispy Pizza–Medium-Sized Italian Sausage, 1 slice	22	2
Thin 'n Crispy Pizza–Medium-Sized Pork Topping, 1 slice	22	2
Thin 'n Crispy Pizza–Medium-Sized Meat Lover's®, 1 slice	22	2
Thin 'n Crispy Pizza–Medium-Sized Veggie Lover's®, 1 slice	24	2
Thin 'n Crispy Pizza–Medium-Sized Pepperoni Lover's®, 1 slice	22	2

	C	F
Thin 'n Crispy Pizza–Medium-Sized Supreme, 1 slice	23	2
Thin 'n Crispy Pizza–Medium-Sized Super Supreme, 1 slice	23	2
Thin 'n Crispy Pizza–Medium-Sized Chicken Supreme, 1 slice	23	2
Pan Pizza–Medium-Sized, 1 slice	28	2
Pan Pizza–Medium-Sized Cheese, 1 slice	29	3
Pan Pizza–Medium-Sized Beef Topping, 1 slice	28	2
Pan Pizza–Medium-Sized Ham, 1 slice	28	2
Pan Pizza–Medium-Sized Pepperoni, 1 slice	29	2
Pan Pizza–Medium-Sized Italian Sausage, 1 slice	29	3
Pan Pizza–Medium-Sized Pork Topping, 1 slice	29	3
Pan Pizza–Medium-Sized Meat Lover's®, 1 slice	30	3
Pan Pizza–Medium-Sized Veggie Lover's®, 1 slice	29	2
Pan Pizza–Medium-Sized Pepperoni Lover's®, 1 slice	29	3
Pan Pizza–Medium-Sized Supreme, 1 slice	30	3
Pan Pizza–Medium-Sized Super Supreme, 1 slice	29	2

Popeye's®

	C	F
Chicken Breast, Mild/Spicy, 1 serving	18	
Chicken Leg, Mild/Spicy, 1 serving	7	
Chicken Thigh, Mild/Spicy, 1 serving	12	
Chicken Wing, Mild/Spicy, 1 serving	10	
Sides: Biscuit, 2 oz, 1 biscuit	25	
Cajun Rice, regular, 1 serving	23	
Cinnamon Apple Turnover, 1 turnover	37	
Coleslaw, regular, 1 serving	20	
Corn on the Cob (1), 1 cob	48	
French Fries, 3 oz, 1 serving	34	
Mashed Potatoes: No Gravy, regular, 1 serving	17	

	C	F
Mashed Potatoes: W. Gravy, regular, 1 serving	18	
Red Beans & Rice, regular, 1 serving	33	

Quizno's Subs®

SANDWICHES

	C	F
Classic Italian Sub: (No Dressing), 1 sandwich	60	
Classic Italian Sub: (No Dressing) small, 9 oz, 1 sandwich	69	
Classic Italian Sub: (No Dressing) Regular, 11½ oz, 1 sandwich	102	
Honey Mustard Chicken w. bacon, large, 22½ oz, 1 sandwich	137	
Philly Cheese Steak, large, 10½ oz, 1 sandwich	92	
Steakhouse Sub (6"), 6½ oz, 1 sandwich	52	
Traditional (no dressing) (8"), 15oz, 1 sandwich	94	
Turkey Ranch Swiss (no dressing), 8", 1 sandwich	89	
Low Fat Sandwiches (small) Honey Bourbon Chicken, 1 sandwich	45	
Low Fat Sandwiches (small) Sierra Smoked Turkey w. Raspberry Chipotle Sauce, 1 sandwich	53	
Low Fat Sandwiches (small) Turkey Lite, 1 sandwich	52	

DRESSINGS

	C	F
Beef Au Jus, 4 oz	3	
Honey Mustard, 2 oz	22	
Italian Vinagarette, 1 oz	3	
Ranch Dressing, 2 oz	3	

SIDES

	C	F
Potato Chips: Classic: Traditional, 1.5 oz, 1 order	25	
Potato Chips: Kettle Cooked, 1.375 oz, 1 order	23	
Potato Chips: Jalapeno, 1.375 oz, 1 order	22	
Potato Chips: Salt & Vinegar, 1.375 oz, 1 order	23	
Potato Chips: Sour Cream & Onion, 1.5 oz, 1 order	25	

DESSERTS

	C	F
Cookies: Peanut Butter, 1 cookie	42	
Cookies: Other, average, 1 cookie	48	

Red Lobster®

DINNER ENTRÉE

	C	F
Atlantic Salmon, 1 serving	0	
Rainbow Trout, 1 serving	0	
Tilapia, 1 serving	0	
Tilapia in a Bag, 1 serving	30	

LUNCH ENTRÉE

	C	F
Atlantic Salmon, 1 serving	0	
Rainbow Trout, 1 serving	2	
Tilapia, 1 serving	0	
Tilapia in a Bag, 1 serving	15	

SPECIALTIES

	C	F
Broiled Flounder, 1 serving	0	
Grilled Chicken, 1 serving	0	
Grilled Shrimp, 1 serving	1	
Jumbo Shrimp Cocktail, 1 serving	2	
King Crab Legs, 1 serving	0	
Live Maine Lobster, 1 serving	2	
Lobster Chops, 1 serving	0	
Rock Lobster, 1 serving	2	
Snow Crab Legs, 1 serving	0	

EXTRAS

	C	F
100% Pure Melted Butter, 1 serving	0	
Baked Potato, no topping, 1 serving	36	
Baked Potato, w/ Pico de Gallo Topping, 1 serving	37	
Cheddar Bay Biscuits, 1 serving	17	
Cocktail Sauce, 1 serving	9	
Fresh Buttered Vegetables, 1 serving	9	
Garden Salad, 1 serving	9	
Jumbo Shrimp Cocktail, 1 serving	1	
King Crab Legs, 1 serving	0	
Lemon Wedge, 1 serving	2	
Maine Lobster Tail, 1 serving	2	
Petite Shrimp Topping, 1 serving	1	
Red Wine Vinaigrette Dressing, 1 serving	5	

	C	F
Seasoned Fresh Broccoli, 1 serving	10	
Snow Crab Legs, 1 serving	0	
Wild Rice Pilaf, 1 serving	36	

Rita's® Water Ice

	C	F
Rita's Cream Ice, kids	44	0
Rita's Cream Ice, regular	70	1
Rita's Cream Ice, large	109	1
Rita's Cream Ice, quart	187	1
Rita's Custard, Kids	32	1
Rita's Custard, regular	43	1
Rita's Custard, large	62	1
Rita's Gelati w/Custard, regular, average	59	0
Rita's Gelati w/Custard, large, average	102	1
Rita's Misto w/Custard, regular, average	90	0
Rita's Misto w/Custard, large average	135	1
Rita's Water Ice, kids	43	0
Rita's Water Ice, regular	69	0
Rita's Water Ice, large	109	0
Rita's Water Ice, quart	185	0

Romano's Macaroni Grill ®

APPETIZERS

	C	F
Calamari Fritti, 1 order	25	2
Chicken Fingerias (fries not included), 1 order	39	1
Mozzarella Alla Caprese, 5 pieces	9	2
Mozzarella Alla Caprese, half order, 3 pieces	5	1
Mozzarella Fritta, 1 order	55	3
Prosciutto Bruschetta, 1 order	67	3
Romano's Sampler - Fried Calamari only, 1 order	9	1
Romano's Sampler - Fried Mozzarella only, 1 order	32	1
Romano's Sampler - Garnish only, 1 order	5	1
Romano's Sampler - Prosciutto Bruschetta only, 1 order	14	1

	C	F
Romano's Sampler - Stuffed Mushrooms only, 1 order	9	1
Romano's Sampler (All 4), 1 order	69	4
Shrimp and Artichoke Dip, 1 order	106	9
Stuffed Mushrooms, 1 order	28	4
Tomato Bruschetta, 1 order	67	7

CHICKEN ENTREES

	C	F
Carmela's Chicken Rigatoni, 1 dinner order	84	6
Carmela's Chicken Rigatoni, 1 lunch order	64	5
Chicken Cannelloni, 1 dinner order	60	4
Chicken Cannelloni, 1 lunch order	40	3
Chicken Marsala, 1 lunch or dinner order, average	78	4
Chicken Parmigiano, 1 dinner order	129	5
Chicken Parmigiano, 1 lunch order	91	4
Chicken Portobello, 1 order	61	5
Chicken Scaloppine, 1 lunch or dinner order, average	67	6
Chicken Toscana, 1 order	12	4
Grilled Chicken & Broccoli, 1 order	49	5
Honey Balsamic Chicken, 1 order	163	14
Pollo Magro Skinny Chicken, 1 order	23	5

OTHER ENTREES

	C	F
Boursin Filet, 1 order	39	5
Eggplant Parmesan, 1 dinner order	118	23
Eggplant Parmesan, 1 lunch order	102	17
Grilled Pork Chops, 1 order	92	8
Mac Grill Grilled Cheese (sandwich only), 1 order	26	0
Mama's Trio, 1 order	110	6
Sausage and Pepper Classico, 1 dinner order	84	9
Sausage and Pepper Classico, 1 lunch order	65	7
Tuscan Ribeye, 1 order	36	5
Veal Marsala, 1 order	119	4
Veal Parmesan, 1 order	116	6
Veal Saltimbocca, 1 order	103	4

PASTAS	C	F
Angelini di Mare, 1 order	88	9
Asiago cream sauce with parmesan over pasta		
Capellini Pomodoro, plain or w/ Chicken, or Shrimp, 1 dinner order, average	112	10
Capellini Pomodoro, plain or w/ Chicken, or Shrimp, 1 lunch order, average	89	8
Cheeseoli, 1 order	39	2
Fettuccine Alfredo, 1 order	50	3
Fettuccine Alfredo, w/ Chicken or Shrimp, 1 lunch or dinner order, average	69	4
Lasagna Bolognese, 1 lunch order	58	5
Lasagna, 1 order	30	3
Lasagna, Twice Baked with Meatballs, 1 order	73	8
Lobster Ravioli, 1 order	55	4
Macaroni 'n Cheese, 1 order	50	2
Mushroom Ravioli, 1 order	41	3
Pasta Milano, 1 dinner order	106	13
Pasta Milano, 1 lunch order	81	10
Penne Arrabbiata, Plain or w/ Chicken or Shrimp, 1 dinner order, average	86	8
Penne Arrabbiata, Plain or w/ Chicken or Shrimp, 1 lunch order, average	66	6
Penne Rustica, 1 dinner order	97	8
Penne Rustica, 1 lunch order	73	6
Spaghetti & Meatballs with Meat or Tomato Sauce, average	56	5
Spaghetti and Meatballs with Meat or Tomato Basil Sauce, 1 lunch order average	87	8
Spaghetti and Meatballs with Meat Sauce, 1 dinner order	206	17
Spaghetti and Meatballs with Tomato Basil Sauce, 1 dinner order	119	11
Spaghetti with Meat Sauce, 1 order	48	4

PIZZA & CALZONES		
BBQ Chicken Pizza, 1 whole	124	6

	C	F
Mona Lisa's Cheese Masterpizza, 1 order	99	1
Mona Lisa's Pepperoni Masterpizza, 1 order	99	6
Pizza Margherita, 1 pizza	112	72
Grilled Chicken Caesar Calzonetto (one whole Calzone)	114	9
Grilled Chicken Caesar Calzonetto, (one Half Calzone)	57	4

SALADS		
Chicken Caesar Salad, 1 salad	26	6
Chicken Florentine Salad with dressing, 1 salad	62	7
Chicken Florentine Salad without dressing, 1 salad	50	7
Insalata Blu (Bleu Salad, accompanies entree), w/ dressing, 1 salad	8	3
Insalata Blu (Bleu Salad), Plain or w/ Chicken w/ dressing, 1 salad	13	5
Insalata Blu (Bleu Salad), Plain or w/ Chicken, w/o dressing, 1 salad	9	5
Insalata Caesar della Casa, 1 salad	13	3
Insalata Garden della Casa w/ or w/o dressing, 1 salad, average	15	3
Insalata Rossa (Red Salad) w/o dressing, 1 salad	17	5
Insalata Rossa (Red Salad) with dressing, 1 salad	34	6
Pasta Salad	35	3
Steak & Arugula Salad, w/ or w/o dressing, average	9	4

DRESSINGS & SAUCES		
Balsamic Vinaigrette Dressing, 2 fl oz	3	0
Caesar Dressing, 2 fl oz	2	0
Creamy Italian Dressing, 2 fl oz	5	0
Fat Free Creamy Italian Dressing, 2 fl oz	5	1
Low Fat Caesar Dressing, 2 fl oz	4	0
Roasted Garlic Lemon Vinaigrette, 2 fl oz	7	0
Strawberry Balsamic Dressing, 2 fl oz	12	1
Toscana Dressing, 2 fl oz	2	0
Basil Aioli Sauce, 2 fl oz	2	0

	C	F
Pizzaiola Sauce, 2 fl oz	4	1

SEAFOOD

	C	F
Grilled Halibut, 1 order	56	2
Grilled Salmon, 1 order	84	5
Mediterranean Shrimp, 1 order	17	4
Mussels Tarantina, 1 order	56	2
Shrimp Diavolo, 1 order	87	8
Shrimp Portofino, 1 lunch or dinner order	66	5
Simple Salmon, 1 order	5	2

SIDES

	C	F
Broccoli Crowns, 4 oz	8	4
Grilled Asparagus, 1 order	4	
Macaroni 'n Cheese (side only)	30	1
Peasant Bread, 1 loaf	85	4
Sauteed Broccoli, 1 order	12	5
Shoestring Fries, 4 oz	27	2

SOUPS

	C	F
Lentil Bean Soup, bowl	48	14
Lentil Bean Soup, cup	24	7
Minestrone Soup, bowl	59	11
Minestrone Soup, cup	39	6
Pasta Fagioli Soup, bowl	88	21
Pasta Fagioli Soup, cup	44	10

DESSERTS

	C	F
Cafe Latte Cheesecake, 1 piece	138	2
Dessert Ravioli, 1 order	214	3
Dessert, 1 order	231	3
Fresh Strawberries (Kid's), 1 order	8	2
Ice Cream Scoop (Kid's), 1 order	43	0
Lemon Passion	151	0
New York Cheesecake (plain), 1 piece	82	0
New York Cheesecake with Caramel Fudge Sauce, 1 piece	168	1
New York Cheesecake with Strawberry Sauce, 1 piece	101	2
Smothered Chocolate Cake, 1 piece	157	6
Strawberries Zabaglione	32	3

	C	F
Tiramisu, 1 order	177	0

Round Table® Pizza

LARGE 14" PIZZA, (PER SLICE, ¹⁄₁₂ OF WHOLE)

	C	F
Chicken & Garlic Gourmet: Pan Crust	39	
Chicken & Garlic Gourmet: Skinny Crust	15	
Chicken Rostadoro: Pan Crust	40	
Chicken Rostadoro: Skinny Crust	20	
Gourmet Veggie: Pan Crust	40	
Gourmet Veggie: Skinny Crust	20	
Hawaiian: Pan Crust	39	
Hawaiian: Skinny Crust 180	20	
Hearty Bacon Supreme: Pan Crust 360	38	
Hearty Bacon Supreme: Skinny Crust	17	
Italian Garlic Supreme: Pan Crust	39	
Italian Garlic Supreme: Skinny Crust	18	
Maui Zaui, Polynesian Sauce: Pan Crust	40	
Maui Zaui, Polynesian Sauce: Skinny Crust	20	
Maui Zaui, Pan Crust	40	
Maui Zaui, Skinny Crust	25	
Montague's All Meat Marvel: Pan Crust	37	
Montague's All Meat Marvel: Skinny Crust	18	
Pepperoni Rostadoro: Pan Crust	40	
Pepperoni Rostadoro: Skinny Crust	21	
Roastin'Toastin' Chicken Club: Pan Crust	39	
Roastin'Toastin' Chicken Club: Skinny Crust	18	
Western BBQ Chicken: Pan Crust	36	
Western BBQ Chicken: Skinny Crust	17	

SANDWICHES

	C	F
Chicken Club	75	
Ham Club	76	
RT Pizza Sandwich	65	
RT Veggie Sandwich	79	

	C	F
Turkey Club	75	

SIDES

	C	F
Buffalo Wings, 6 pieces	2	
Garlic Bread, 4.6 oz	59	
Garlic Bread with Cheese, 6.6 oz	59	
Honey BBQ Wings, 6 pieces	8	

Roy Rogers®

	C	F
Big Country Breakfast: w. Bacon	61	
Big Country Breakfast: w. Sausage	61	
Big Country Breakfast: w. Ham	67	
Hamburger	33	
Cheeseburger	34	
Hamburger, ¼ lb	41	
Cheeseburger, ¼ lb	42	
Sourdough Grilled Chicken	46	
Roast Beef Sandwich	30	
Chicken Fillet Sandwich	49	
Grilled Chicken Sandwich	32	
Fries, regular	49	
Fries, large	59	
Hot Fudge Sundae	50	

Ruby Tuesday®

APPETIZERS (PER HALF ORDER, SAUCES NOT INCLUDED)

	C	F
Asian Glazed Wings	7	
Asian Steamed Dumplings	13	
Blackened Crabcakes	3	
Cheesy Spinach Dip	19	
Chili Queso Fries	31	
Crispy Buffalo Wontons	10	
Dble Cheese/Chkn Quesadilla, average	13	
Jumb'o'Rings	26	
Kickin' Queso	23	
Loaded Cheese Fries	29	
Mega Nachos	34	
Original Super Sampler	39	

	C	F
Say Cheese Sticks	13	
Southwestern Spring Rolls	15	
Spicy Buffalo Wings	2	
Texas Straws	27	
Tuesday Tenders, Classic	9	

BURGERS

	C	F
Burgers: American Cheeseburger	53	
Bacon Cheeseburger	53	
Chili Cheeseburger, no sides	56	
Crispy Chicken Club, no sides	54	
Killer Fish, no sides	43	
Lulu's Turkey, no sides	42	
Macho Nacho, no sides	47	
Mama Mia, no sides	57	
Plain Jane, no sides	53	
Ruby's Chicken, no sides	49	
Ruby's Sliders, no sides	74	
Surf & Turf, no sides	54	
Ultimate Colossal	81	
Veggie	66	

SPECIALTIES (SIDES NOT INCLUDED)

	C	F
Big Island Shrimp	103	
Blackened Crabcakes	68	
Chesapeake Catch	54	
Creole Catch	44	
Louisiana Fried Shrimp	120	
New Orleans Seafood	48	
Stacker: Chopped Steak	89	
Sirloin Tips, full pound	92	

PASTAS: PER ORDER (GARLIC TOAST NOT INCLUDED)

	C	F
Baked Chicken & Broccoli	126	
Baked Roma Chicken	110	
Chicken Parmesan	127	
Original Sonora	120	
Shrimp Alfredo Pasta	111	

STEAKS & MORE (SIDES NOT INCLUDED)

	C	F
Peppercorn Mushroom Sirloin	9	

	C	F
Petitie Sirloin	1	
Ragin'Cajun Ribeye	6	
Ruby's Ribeye	4	
Sirloin Tips, Full rack	7	
Steak & Cake Combo	13	
Steak & Coconut Shrimp Combo	23	
Top Sirloin	1	
Triple Play Platter	104	
Tuesday Tenders: Classic	76	
Tuesday Tenders: Spicy Buffalo	82	

HANG OFF THE PLATE RIBS: (PER ORDER, NO SAUCE)

	C	F
Asian/Classic/Spicy, Full Rack	95	
Asian/Classic/Spicy, Half Rack	81	
Memphis Dry Rub, Full Rack	73	
Memphis Dry Rub, Half Rack	70	

SAUCES & DRESSINGS (PER 7 OZ)

	C	F
Barbecue See/Sweet & Hot Ginger Sauce	13	
Bleu Cheese Dressing	1	
Caesar Dressing	2	
Cocktail See; Strawberry Sauce, average	7	
Honey Mustard Dressing	5	
Marinara Sauce	2	
Ranch Dressing	1	
Ranch Light Dressing	1	
Remoulade	1	
Smoky Honey Dijon Dressing	7	
Sour Cream	2	

SIDES & SALADS

	C	F
Salads: Caesar	5	
Salads: Carolina Chicken, no sides	38	
Baked Potato w. Butter & Sour Cream	62	
Brown Rice Pilaf w. Cheese & Tomato	36	
Coleslaw	12	
Creamy Mashed Cauliflower	15	
Steamed Broccoli in Buttery Sauce	8	
Jumb'o'Rings	42	

	C	F
Ruby's Mashed Potatoes	55	
Ruby's Million Dollar Fries	54	
Sauteed Mushrooms	4	
Texas Straws	54	

SOUPS

	C	F
Baked French Onion	29	
Broccoli & Cheese	15	
White Chicken Chili	28	

DESSERTS

	C	F
Blondie	104	
Brownie	146	
Chocolate Tallcake	130	
Ice Cream Pie	110	
Low Carb Cheesecake	6	

Ruby's Diner®

	C	F
Chicken RubyBurger–Special Request (without added salt, margarine or mayo), 1 burger	41	
Chinese Chicken Salad–Special Request (no added salt or sesame dressing), 1 salad	21	
Fresh Roast Turkey Breast Sandwich–Special Request (without margarine or mayo), 1 sandwich	41	
Skinny Fries (request no added salt), 1 order	38	
Soft Veggie Tacos–Special Request (request less cheese, salsa–not dressing)	67	
Turkey RubyBurger–Special Request (without added salt, margarine or RubySauce), 1 burger	43	
Veggie RubyBurger (request no added salt, margarine or RubySauce), 1 burger	64	

Saladworks ®

SALADS

	C	F
Bently Salad, 1	7	3
BLT Salad, 1	8	3
Caesar Salad, 1	18	3

	C	F
Chicken Caesar Salad, 1	18	3
Dorte Salad, 1	180	9
Garden Deluxe Salad, 1	134	15
Garden Salad, 1	15	5
Greek Salad, 1	11	4
Mandarin Chicken Salad, 1	59	7
Newport Salad, 1	7	3
Nicoise Salad, 1	101	7
Pastizza Salad, 1	174	9
Shrimp Caesar Salad, 1	18	3
Spensa Salad, 1	204	17
Spinach Salad, 1	19	3
Sunnio Salad, 1	202	16
Tivoli Salad, 1	102	6
Tuna Pasta Salad, 1	173	9
Turkey Club Salad, 1	101	6

DRESSINGS

	C	F
Balsamic Vinaigrette Dressing, 28 g	3	0
Blue Cheese Dressing, 28 g	2	0
Creamy Italian Dressing, 28 g	1	0
Dijon Honey Mustard Dressing, 28 g	2	0
Fat Free Balsamic Dressing, 28 g with Sundried Tomato	3	0
Fat Free Caesar Dressing, 28 g	3	0
Fat Free Vinaigrette Dressing, 28 g	2	0
French Dressing, 28 g	6	0
Green Goddess Dressing, 28 g	2	0
Herbal Ranch Dressing, 28 g	3	0
Low Fat Creamy Italian Dressing, 28 g	2	0
Low Fat Dijon Honey Mustard Dressing, 28 g	2	0
Royal Caesar Dressing, 28 g	0	0
Vinaigrette Italian Dressing, 28 g	4	0

Sbarro's®

ENTREES (PER SERVING)

	C
Baked Ziti w. Sauce	43
Chicken Parmigiana	16
Meat Lasagne	36
Spaghetti w. Sauce	120

PIZZA (PER SLICE)	C	F
Cheese	60	
Pepperoni	61	
Sausage	60	
Supreme	63	

STUFFED PIZZA (PER SLICE)

	C
Spinach & Broccoli	89
Pepperoni	89

Schlotzsky's®

BREADS/BUNS

	C
Dark Rye, regular	68
Sourdough, regular	66
Wheat, regular	66
Jalapeno Cheese, regular	66
Pizza Crust	68

ORIGINAL SANDWICHES (PER SANDWICH)

	C
The Original, regular	79
Large Original, family size	152
Deluxe Original, regular	84
Ham & Cheese Original, regular	82
Turkey Original, regular	81

SANDWICHES (PER REGULAR SANDWICH)

	C
Albacore Tuna	77
Albacore Tuna Melt	83
BLT	70
Chicken Breast	80
Chicken Club	75
Corned Beef	78
Corned Beef Reuben	82
Dijon Chicken	74
Fiesta Chicken	79
Pastrami & Swiss	81
Pastrami Reuben	83
Pesto Chicken	73
Roast Beef	78
Roast Beef & Cheese	83
Santa Fe Chicken	81

	C	F
Smoked Turkey Breast	75	
Texas Schlotzsky's	76	
The Philly	86	
The Vegetarian	79	
Turkey & Bacon Club	79	
Turkey Guacamole	84	
Turkey Reuben	80	
Vegetable Club	76	
Western Vegetarian	76	
Wraps: Asian Almond Chicken	72	
Chicken Caesar	40	
Salsa Chicken w.Cheddar	44	
Zesty Albacore Tuna	45	

SOUPS: PER CUP (8 OZ)

	C	F
Boston Clam Chowder	24	
Broccoli Cheese w. Florets	23	
Chicken Gumbo	13	
Chicken Tortilla	13	
Chicken w. Wild Rice	36	
Minestrone	17	
Old-Fashioned Chicken Noodle	18	

DELI SALADS (PER 5 OZ CONTAINER)

	C	F
Albacore Tuna, small, 4.4 oz	2	
California Pasta	10	
Elbow Macaroni	23	
Homestyle Cole Slaw	24	
Mustard Potato	31	
Potato	35	

LEAF SALADS (W/OUT DRESSING/ CROUTONS/NOODLES)

	C	F
Chicken Caesar	4	
Chinese Chicken	10	
Garden Salad	7	
Greek Salad	10	
Ham & Turkey Chefs	13	
Smoked Turkey Chefs	3	

PIZZAS (8")

	C	F
Bacon, Tomato & Mushroom	78	
Barbeque Chicken	93	
Chicken & Pesto, New Orleans	78	
Double Cheese	76	
Double Cheese & Pepperoni	77	
Fresh Tomato & Pesto	76	
Mediterranean	72	
Smoked Turkey & Jalapeno	80	
Thai Chicken	89	
The Original Combination	79	
Vegetarian Special	76	

SALAD EXTRAS

	C	F
Chow Mein Noodles	9	
Garlic Chinese Croutons, ½ oz, pkg	5	
Greek Balsamic Vinaigrette, 1.5 oz	2	
Light Italian Dressing, 1.5 oz	3	
Olde World Caesar Dress., 1.5 oz	1	
Ranch Dressing: Traditional, 1.5 oz	1	
Ranch Dressing: Spicy, 1.5 oz	2	
Ranch Dressing: Light Spicy, 1.5 oz	9	
Schlotzsky's Deli Chips, 1.5 oz bag	26	
Sesame Ginger Vinaigrette, 1.5 oz	8	
Thousand Island Dressing, 1.5 oz	6	

KID'S DEALS (WITHOUT COOKIE OR DRINK)

	C	F
Cheese Pizza	72	
Cheese Sandwich	49	
PBJ Sandwich	71	
Pepperoni Pizza	72	

DESSERTS & COOKIES

	C	F
Fudge Brownie	46	
Cookies: Oatmeal Raisin	24	
Cookies w. Real M&M's	20	
Other cookie varieties, average	23	
Cheesecake: Cookies & Creme	36	
Cheesecake: New York; Strawberry Swirl	31	

Shoney's®

BREAKFAST	C	F
All Star Breakfast, no extras	1	
Deluxe Pancake Platter	300	
Half Stack Pancake Platter	187	
Big Eater Steak Breakfast, no extras	1	
Country Fried Steak Breakfast	49	
Sunrise Breakfast	88	
Sausage Biscuit (1)	42	

BURGERS	C	F
Ail-American: Burger or Bacon Cheeseburger	44	
Mushroom Swiss Burger	49	
Famous Patty Melt	40	
Half 0-Pound Burger	130	

SANDWICHES	C	F
Blackened Chicken	122	
Charbroiled Chicken Sandwich	122	
Chicken Parmesan Sandwich	80	
Corned Beef Reuben	37	
Fish Sandwich	126	
Fried Chicken Sandwich	76	
Original Slim Jim Sandwich	122	
Raymond's French Dip	53	
Turkey Club/Whole Wheat	46	
Ultimate Grilled Cheese S'wich	77	

STEAKS	C	F
BBQ Ribs	124	
Choice Sirloin, 6 oz	127	
Half-0-Pound w. Grilled Onions	133	
Half-0-Pound w. Grilled Mushr.	127	
Ribeye, 8oz	127	
Southwest Half-0-Pound	83	
T-Bone, 12 oz	127	

SURF & TURF	C	F
Ribeye & 5 Fried Shrimp	138	
Ribeye & 6 Grilled Shrimp	128	
Sirloin & 5 Fried Shrimp	138	
Sirloin & 6 Grilled Shrimp	128	

	C	F
T-Bone & 5 Fried Shrimp	138	
T-Bone & 6 Grilled Shrimp	128	

RIB COMBOS (WITH FRIES)	C	F
¼ Rack & BBQ Chicken	103	
¼ Rack & Tenderloins	120	
¼ Rack & Fried Shrimp	113	
¼ Rack & Grilled Shrimp	103	

BLUE PLATE SPECIALS	C	F
Cajun Whitefish	56	
Baked Whitefish	58	
Grandma's Meatloaf w. Glaze	92	
Grandma's Meatloaf w. Gravy	87	
Original Country Fried Steak	103	
Grilled Liver & Onions	79	
Ham Steak Dinner (no veges)	60	
Roast Beef Platter (no veges)	96	

PASTA (PER SERVING)	C	F
Chicken Alfredo	170	
Italian Feast	204	
Pasta Ya-Ya	176	
Shrimp Alfredo	171	
Spaghetti	63	

SEAFOOD	C	F
Fish 'n' Shrimp	129	
Fried Fish Platter	122	
Grilled Cod/Salmon Lite	0	
Grilled Salmon	95	
Grilled Shrimp	95	
Grilled Shrimp Lite	30	
Shrimper's Feast	127	
Shrimp Stir Fry	131	

SIDES	C	F
Baked Potato, Plain	67	
French Fries, 4 oz	25	
Onion Rings, 1 order (7 rings)	83	

CHICKEN	C	F
Chicken Stir Fry	172	
Charbroiled Blackened Chicken	100	
Charbroiled Chicken Breast	99	
Fried Chicken Tenderloins	121	
Monterey Chicken	83	
Smothered Chicken	90	

JUNIOR MEALS		
Fish 'N Chips	29	
Chicken Dinner	12	

DESSERTS, ICE CREAM		
Apple Pie: a la Mode	173	
Apple Pie: a la Mode w/ NutraSweet	64	
Cheesecake, 1 slice, 4 oz	23	
Hot Fudge Sundae	75	
Original Strawberry Pie, 1 slice	45	
Ultimate Hot Fudge Sundae	75	
Cherry/Peach Pie w. NutraSweet	68	
Caramel Sundae	83	
Chocolate Milk Shake	141	
Strawberry Sundae	85	
Walnut Brownie a la Mode	60	

Skippers Seafood & Chowder®

ENTREES		
Clam Strips, 1 order	39	6
Fish Bites (12 Pieces) & Chips, 1 order	107	6
Fish Bites (18 Pieces) & Chips, 1 order	143	9
Fish Bites (6 Pieces) & Chips, 1 order	94	7
Fish Sandwich (1)	105	4
Fried Chicken Sandwich (1)	117	3
Grilled Chicken Breast, 1 order	0	0
Grilled Chicken Sandwich w/ chips (ff) & coleslaw, 1 order	92	3
Grilled Halibut, 1 order	0	0
Grilled Salmon, 1 order	0	0
Halibut, 1 order	51	0
Homestyle Chicken Tenderloin (1 tenderloin)	13	0

	C	F
Original Fish Fillet (1 fillet)	12	1
Original Fish, 2 pieces, w/chips (ff) & kids side	59	2
Original Fish, 3 pieces, w/chips (ff) & kids side	71	3
Original Fish, 4 pieces, w/chips (ff) & kids side	83	4
Original Shrimp, 9 pieces	36	1

BASKET ENTREES		
Clam Strip Seafood, 1 basket	113	12
Clams & Fish Combination, 1 basket	91	8
Popcorn Shrimp Seafood, (1) basket, w/chips (ff) & kids side	96	2
Prawn & Fish Seafood, (1) basket, w/chips (ff) & kids side	61	2
Prawn Seafood, (1) basket, w/chips (ff) & kids side	52	0
Shrimp & Fish Combination, (1) basket, w/chips (ff) & kids side	83	2
Shrimp Seafood, (1) basket (original recipe), w/chips (ff) & kids side	107	3
Shrimp Trio Seafood, (1) basket, w/chips (ff) & kids side	123	4

KIDS		
Kids Catch Chicken Tenderloin, w/chips (ff) & kids side, 1 order	79	1
Kids Catch Fish Bites, w/chips (ff) & kids side, 1 order	84	3
Kids Catch Grilled Cheese Sandwich, w/chips (ff) & kids side, 1 order	97	3
Kids Catch Shrimp, w/chips (ff) & kids side, 1 order	91	2
Skippers Platter, w/chips (ff) & kids side, 1 order	122	8

SALADS		
Large Caesar Salad (1)	17	4
Large Caesar Salad w/Chicken or Salmon, 1 salad	12	2
Large Green Salad (1)	10	2
Small Caesar Salad, Plain or w/chicken or salmon, 1 salad	8	2
Small Green Salad, no dressing, (1)	5	2

SIDES	C	F
Baked Potato, 1 plain	48	5
Coleslaw, 1 Bowl	29	0
Coleslaw, 1 Cup	9	0
Coleslaw, small, 1 order	7	0
French Fries, 1 order	27	0
French Fries, family size (feeds 4)	122	12
Grilled Veggies, 1 order	8	3
Hush Puppies, 12 pieces	187	14
Hush Puppies, 3 pieces	47	3
Hush Puppies, 6 pieces	94	7

SOUPS	C	F
Clam Chowder, 1 bowl	23	1
Clam Chowder, 1 cup	14	0

Sonic Drive-In®

BURGERS & SANDWICHES	C
#1. Burger w. Mayonnaise	43
#2. Burger w. Mustard	43
#1 . Cheeseburger w. Mayonnaise	44
#2. Cheeseburger w. Mustard	44
Bacon Cheeseburger	44
Super Sonic # 1 w. Mayonnaise	45
Super Sonic # 2 w. Mustard	46
Junior Burger	27
Bacon Cheddar Burger Toasted Sandwich	60
Chicken Club Toasted Sandwich	75
Breaded Chicken Sandwich	66
Grilled Chicken Sandwich	31

CHICKEN ENTREES & WRAPS	C
Chicken Strip, w. Ranch Dressing Wrap	55
Grilled Chicken w. Ranch Dressing Wrap	40
Chicken Strip Dinner	86
Chicken Strip Snack	22
Jumbo Popcorn Chicken: large	36
Jumbo Popcorn Chicken: Snack	24

SALADS	C
Salads: Grilled Chicken, no dressing	20

	C	F
Jumbo Popcorn Chicken, no dressing	39	
Santa Fe Grilled Chicken, no dressing	33	

CONEYS	C
Plain: regular	23
Plain: Extra Long	44
Cheese: regular	24
Cheese: Extra-Long	47
Corn Dog	23

BREAKFAST	C
Breakfast Burrito	36
Bacon Egg & Cheese Toaster	40
Sausage Egg & Cheese Toaster	44
Ham Egg & Cheese Toaster	41
Sonic Sunrise Breakfast: regular	60
Sonic Sunrise Breakfast: large	100

FAVES & CRAVES	C
French Fries: regular, 3.7 oz	22
French Fries: large, 4.9 oz	30
Super Sonic, 7.2 oz	44
Ched'R'Peppers (4)	29
Cheese Fries: regular, 4.3 oz	23
Cheese Fries: large, 5.5 oz	31
Chili Cheese Fries: regular, 5.1 oz	24
Mozzarella Sticks, 5.4 oz	35
Onion Rings: regular	66
Onion Rings: large, 19 oz	102
Onion Rings: Super Sonic, 20.6 oz	141
Tater Tots: regular, 4.2 oz	27
Tater Tots: large, 6.1 oz	40
Tater Tots: Supersonic, 8.1 oz	53
Cheese Tater Tots: regular	28
Cheese Tater Tots: large, 6.8 oz	41
Chili Cheese Tater Tots: regular	28
Chili Cheese Tater Tots: large, 9 oz	43

DESSERTS	C
Banana Split, 12.5 oz	75
Chocolate Sundae, 8.5 oz	41
Dish of Vanilla, 7 oz	19

	C	F
Hot Fudge Sundae, 8.5 oz	40	
Ice cream Cone	23	
Pineapple Sundae, 9 oz	53	
Strawberry Sundae	32	

DRINKS

	C	F
Barq's Root Beer, large	90	
Coca-Cola, large	81	
Coca-Cola Float, large	59	
Blasts: regular, all types, average	58	
Blasts: large, all types, average	89	
Slushes: small, average	58	
Slushes: regular, average, all flavors	81	
Slushes: large, average, all flavors	127	
Wacky Pack, average	50	
Route 44, average	123	
Slush Floats / Cream Slush: regular, average	52	
Slush Floats / Cream Slush: large, average	74	

Souplantation®

SOUPS (PER 1 CUP)

	C	F
Low Fat: Chicken Tortilla	5	
Low Fat: Minestrone	20	
Low Fat: Vegetable Medley	14	
Regular: Chesapeake Corn Chowder	30	
Regular: Cream of Mushroom	15	
Regular: Irish Potato Leek	23	
Regular: Manhattan Clam Chowder	16	
Regular: Minestrone w. Italian Sausage	14	
Regular: Navy Bean w. Ham	30	
Regular: Vegetarian Harvest	23	
Chili: Low-Fat Kettle House	26	

BREADS & SALADS

	C	F
Breads: Sourdough	27	
Breads: Buttermilk Cornbread, 1 piece	27	
Focaccia: Garlic Parmesan	15	
Focaccia: Pizza /Tomatillo	16	

	C	F
Antipasto Salad; BBQ, average, per 1 cup	6	
Caesar Salad Asiago, average, per 1 cup	10	
Won Ton Chicken Happiness, average, per 1 cup	12	

PREPARED SALADS (PER ½ CUP)

	C	F
Aunt Doris' Red Pepper Slaw	18	
Baja Bean & Cilantro	29	
BBQ Potato	20	
Carrot Raisin	17	
Dijon Potato w. Garlic Dill Vinegar	9	
Greek Couscous w. Feta Cheese	19	
Oriental Ginger Slaw w. Krab	8	
Southern Dill Potato	20	
Thai Noodle w. Peanut Sauce	17	
Zesty Tortellini	18	

DRESSINGS & CROUTONS (PER 2 TBSP)

	C	F
Blue Cheese Dressing	3	
Balsamic Vinaigrette	1	
Italian Dressing	1	
Italian Dressing Fat Free	5	
Honey Mustard Dressing	8	
Honey Mustard Dressing Fat Free	10	
Ranch Dressing	1	
Ranch Dressing Fat Free	2	
Thousand Island Dressing	3	
Croutons, Garlic Parmesan, 5 pieces	2	

HOT TOSSED PASTAS (PER 1 CUP)

	C	F
Bruschetta	41	
Creamy Bruschetta	43	
Garden Vegetable: w. Meatballs	42	
Garden Vegetable: w. Italian Sausage	42	
Italian Vegetable Beef	43	
Vegetarian Marinara w. Basil	44	

MUFFINS

	C	F
Chocolate Brownie	22	
Georgia Peach Poppyseed	20	
Tangy Lemon	24	

	C	F
Wildly Blue Blueberry, small	22	
Fruit Medley Bran	17	

DESSERTS

	C	F
Apple Cobbler, ½ Cup	64	
Apple Medley (fat-free), ½ cup	18	
Banana Royale (fat-free), ½ cup	20	
Chocolate Chip Cookie, small	10	
Chocolate Lava Cake, ½ cup	56	
Jell-o, flavored, ½ cup	20	
Rice Pudding, ½ cup	20	
Vanilla Pudding, ½ cup	24	
Chocolate Syrup, 2 tbsp	18	
Granola Topping, 2 tbsp	16	
Soft Serve: Chocolate,½ cup	21	
Soft Serve: Vanilla (reduced fat), ½ cup	22	

Steak Escape®

SMALL 7" SANDWICHES (NO CHEESE OR CONDIMENTS)

	C	F
Grand Gobbler	67	
Grand Escape	64	
Grandest Chicken	64	
Great Escape	63	
Hambrosia	69	
Ragin' Cajun	63	
Turkey Club	65	
Vegetarian	64	
Wild West BBQ	72	

LARGE 12" SANDWICHES (NO CHEESE OR CONDIMENTS)

	C	F
Grand Gobbler	116	
Grand Escape	110	
Grandest Chicken	108	
Great Escape	119	
Hambrosia	108	
Ragin' Cajun	111	
Turkey Club	109	
Vegetarian	126	
Wild West BBQ		

FRESH SALADS (NO CHEESE OR CONDIMENTS)

	C	F
Side Salad	8	
Grilled Salad: w/ Chicken	11	
Grilled Salad: w/ Ham	8	
Grilled Salad: w/ Steak	11	
Grilled Salad: w/ Turkey	8	

POTATOES & FRIES

	C	F
Smashed, Plain, 14 oz	53	
Smashed, w/ Chicken, 14 oz	56	
Smashed, w/ Ham, 14 oz	59	
Smashed, w/ Steak, 14 oz	56	
Smashed, w/ Turkey, 14 oz	59	
Smashed, Loaded w/ Bacon & Cheddar	91	
Smashed, Loaded w/ Ranch & Bacon	87	
Fresh Cut Fries: small, 6 oz	67	
Fresh Cut Fries: medium, 7.8 oz	87	
Fresh Cut Fries: large, 11.3 oz	123	
Fresh Cut Fries: Loaded: Bacon & Cheddar	88	
Fresh Cut Fries: Ranch & Bacon	84	

CONDIMENTS

	C	F
Mayonnaise, 1 oz	0	
BBQ Sauce, 1 oz	9	
Cheddar Cheese, 1 oz	1	

Starbucks®

	C	F
Americano, 1 each	3	0
Latte, Whole Milk, 1 each	22	0
Latte, 2% Fat Milk, 1 each	22	0
Latte, Nonfat Milk, 1 each	23	0
Latte, Soy Milk, 1 each	10	5
Latte, Breve (half & half), 1 each	16	0
Mocha, Whole Milk, 1 each	40	2
Mocha, 2% Fat Milk, 1 each	40	2
Mocha, Nonfat Milk, 1 each	40	2
Mocha, Soymilk, 1 each	44	4
Vanilla Syrup, 1 each	21	0
Hazelnut Syrup, 1 each	21	0

	C	F
Mocha Syrup, 1 each	24	2
Caramel Sauce, 1 each	2	0
Sweetened Whipped Cream Topping, 1 each	2	0
Power Packet, 1 each	23	1
Mocha, Breve (half & half), 1 each	36	2
Cappuccino, Whole Milk, 1 each	15	0
Cappuccino, 2% Fat Milk, 1 each	15	0
Cappuccino, Nonfat Milk, 1 each	15	0
Cappuccino, Soy Milk, 1 each	7	4
Caramel Macchiato, Whole Milk, 1 each	36	0
Caramel Macchiato, 2% Fat Milk, 1 each	36	0
Caramel Macchiato, Nonfat Milk, 1 each	36	0
Caramel Macchiato, Soy Milk, 1 each	44	2
Caramel Macchiato, Breve (half & half), 1 each	37	0
Eggnog Latte, Whole Milk, 1 each	49	0
Eggnog Latte, Nonfat Milk, 1 each	49	0
Espresso Solo, 1 each	1	0
Espresso Doppio, 1 each	2	0
Dipping Sauces: Buffalo Sauce ¾ oz, 1 each	49	2
Steamed Cider, 1 each	57	0
Tazo Chai, 1 each	52	0
White Chocolate Mocha, Whole Milk, 1 each	60	0
White Chocolate Mocha, 2% Fat Milk, 1 each	61	0
White Chocolate Mocha, Nonfat Milk, 1 each	61	0
White Chocolate Mocha, Soymilk, 1 each	65	2
White Chocolate Mocha, Breve, 1 each	56	0
White Hot Chocolate, 1 each	63	0
Iced Cafe Americano, 1 each	3	0
Iced Café Latte, Whole Milk, 1 each	13	0
Iced Café Latte, 2% Fat Milk, 1 each	14	0
Iced Café Latte, Nonfat Milk, 1 each	14	0
Iced Café Latte, Soy Milk, 1 each	6	3

	C	F
Iced Café Mocha, Whole Milk, 1 each	36	2
Iced Tazo Chai, Whole Milk, 1 each	66	0
Iced White Chocolate Mocha, Whole Milk, 1 each	52	0
Frappuccino®, Caramel, 1 each	61	0
Frappuccino®, Chocolate Brownie, 1 each	88	2
Frappuccino®, Coffee, 1 each	55	0
Frappuccino®, Eggnog, 1 each	57	0
Frappuccino®, Espresso, 1 each	46	0
Frappuccino®, Mocha, 1 each	61	0
TazoBerry®, 1 each	53	0
TazoBerry® & Cream, 1 each	63	0
Short Size Drinks equal 8 oz, 1 each		
Tall Size Drinks equal 12 oz, 1 each		
Grande Size Drinks equal 16 oz, 1 each		

Subway®

	C	F
6", Low Fat Sandwich, Ham, 1 each	47	4
6", Low Fat Sandwich, Oven Roasted Chicken Breast, 1 each	47	4
6", Low Fat Sandwich, Roast Beef, 1 each	45	4
6", Low Fat Sandwich, Turkey Breast, 1 each	46	4
6", Low Fat Sandwich, Turkey Breast & Ham, 1 each	47	4
6", Low Fat Sandwich, Subway Club®, 1 each	47	4
6", Low Fat Sandwich, Sweet Onion Chicken Teriyaki, 1 each	59	4
6", Low Fat Sandwich, Veggie Delite®, 1 each	44	4
6", Regular Sandwich, Cheese Steak, 1 each	47	5
6", Regular Sandwich, Chicken & Bacon Ranch, 1 each	47	5
6", Regular Sandwich, Chicken Parmesan, 1 each	64	5
6", Regular Sandwich, Chipotle Southwest Cheese Steak, 1 each	48	6
6", Regular Sandwich, Tuna, 1 each	45	4

	C	F
6", Regular Sandwich, Cold Cut Combo, 1 each	47	4
6", Regular Sandwich, Italian BMT®, 1 each	47	4
6", Regular Sandwich, Meatball Marinara, 1 each	63	7
6", Regular Sandwich, Spicy Italian, 1 each	46	4
6", Regular Sandwich, Subway Melt®, 1 each	48	4
Deli Style Sandwiches, Tuna (with cheese), 1 each	35	3
Deli Style Sandwiches, Ham, 1 each	36	3
Deli Style Sandwiches, Roast Beef, 1 each	35	3
Deli Style Sandwiches, Turkey Breast, 1 each	36	3
Wraps, Chicken & Bacon Ranch (with cheese), 1 each	18	9
Wraps, Tuna (with cheese), 1 each	16	9
Wraps, Turkey Breast & Bacon Melt (w/Chipotle Sauce), 1 each	20	9
Wraps, Turkey Breast, 1 each	18	9
Salads, Grilled Chicken & Baby Spinach, (w/o dressings or croutons), 1 each	11	4
Salads, Subway Club®, (w/o dressings or croutons), 1 each	15	4
Salads, Tuna (with cheese), (w/o dressings or croutons), 1 each	12	4
Salads, Veggie Delite®, (w/o dressings or croutons), 1 each	12	4
Dipping Sauces: Buffalo Sauce ¾ oz, 1 each	1	0
Salad Dressings, Fat Free Italian, 1 each	7	0
Salad Dressings, Ranch (.5 net carb), 1 each	1	0.5
6" Double Meat Sandwich, Turkey Breast, 1 each	48	4
6" Double Meat Sandwich, Turkey Breast & Ham, 1 each	50	4
6" Double Meat Sandwich, Ham, 1 each	57	4
6" Double Meat Sandwich, Roast Beef, 1 each	46	4

	C	F
6" Double Meat Sandwich, Subway Club®, 1 each	50	4
6" Double Meat Sandwich, Oven Roasted Chicken, 1 each	50	4
6" Double Meat Sandwich, Classic Tuna, 1 each	45	4
6" Double Meat Sandwich, Seafood Sensation, 1 each	58	5
6" Double Meat Sandwich, Italian BMT®, 1 each	49	4
6" Double Meat Sandwich, Cold Cut Combo, 1 each	49	4
6" Double Meat Sandwich, Turkey Breast, Ham & Bacon Melt, 1 each	51	4
6" Double Meat Sandwich, Cheese Steak, 1 each	50	6
6" Double Meat Sandwich, Meatball Marinara, 1 each	82	10
6" Double Meat Sandwich, Sweet Onion Chick. Teriyaki, 1 each	68	4
6" Double Meat Sandwich, Chipotle Southwest Cheese Steak, 1 each	51	7
6" limited time offer, Absolute Angus Steak, 1 each	44	4
6" limited time offer, Barbecue Rib Patty, 1 each	47	4
6" limited time offer, Barbecue Chicken, 1 each	52	5
6" limited time offer, BBQ Steak & Monterey Cheddar Cheese, 1 each	53	6
6" limited time offer, Big Hot Pastrami/Extreme Toasted Pastrami, 1 each	48	4
6" limited time offer, Buffalo Chicken, 1 each	46	5
6" limited time offer, Chipotle Chicken & Bacon Double Cheese Melt, 1 each	47	5
6" limited time offer, Gardenburger®, 1 each	66	9
6" limited time offer, Garlic Lover's Roast Beef Double Cheese Melt, 1 each	48	5
6" limited time offer, Pastrami, 1 each	49	5

Taco Bell®

	C	F
Chalupa Supreme™–Chicken, 1 serving	28	2
Chalupa Supreme™–Steak, 1 serving	27	2
Chalupa Baja™–Beef, 1 serving	30	3
Chalupa Baja™–Chicken, 1 serving	28	2
Chalupa Baja™–Steak, 1 serving	27	2
Chalupa Nacho Cheese–Beef, 1 serving	30	3
Chalupa Nacho Cheese–Chicken, 1 serving	29	2
Chalupa Nacho Cheese–Steak, 1 serving	28	1
Gordita Supreme®–Beef, 1 serving	27	3
Gordita Supreme®–Chicken, 1 serving	28	3
Gordita Supreme®–Steak, 1 serving	27	3
Gordita Baja™–Beef, 1 serving	29	4
Gordita Baja™–Chicken, 1 serving	28	3
Gordita Baja™–Steak, 1 serving	28	3
Gordita Nacho Cheese–Beef, 1 serving	30	4
Gordita Nacho Cheese–Chicken, 1 serving	29	3
Gordita Nacho Cheese–Steak, 1 serving	28	2
Cheesy Gordita Crunch, 1 serving	44	6
Cheesy Gordita Crunch Supreme, 1 serving	47	6
Nachos, 1 serving	34	3
Nachos Supreme™, 1 serving	44	9
Nachos BellGrande®, 1 serving	83	17
Mucho Grande Nachos, 1 serving	116	18
Pintos'n Cheese, 1 serving	18	10
Mexican Rice, 1 serving	23	<1
Cinnamon Twists, 1 serving	27	<1
Zesty Chicken Border Bowl w/ Dressing, 1 serving	58	10
Zesty Chicken Border Bowl w/o Dressing, 1 serving	55	10
Tostada, 1 serving	27	11
Mexican Pizza, 1 serving	42	8

	C	F
Enchirito®–Beef, 1 serving	33	9
Enchirito®–Chicken, 1 serving	32	7
Enchirito®–Steak, 1 serving	31	7
MexiMelt®, 1 serving	22	4
Taco Salad with Salsa, 1 serving	69	16
Taco Salad with Salsa without Shell, 1 serving	31	15
Cheese Quesadilla, 1 serving	39	4
Chicken Quesadilla, 1 serving	40	4

TCBY®

FROZEN YOGURT (PER ½ CUP, NO TOPPINGS)

	C
96% Fat Free Yogurt	23
Low Carb Yogurt	16
Non fat Yogurt	23
Non fat No Sugar Added Yogurt	20

ICE CREAMS (PER 2.5 OZ, NO TOPPINGS)

	C
Hand-Dipped: Butter Pecan	14
Chocolate	15
Chocolate Chip	15
Chunck	16
Cookie Dough, Pralines & Cream	17
Mint Chocolate Chip	15
Pistachio	13
Rocky Road	20
Strawberry	13
Vanilla, White Chocolate Caramel	13

CONES & SORBET

	C
Sugar or Junior Waffle	15
Waffle Cone	22
Non fat & Nondairy Sorbet	24

SMOOTHIES (PER SMALL - 20 FL.OZ)

	C
A Lotta Colada	69
A Lotta Colada w. yogurt	99
Berry Slim	75
Berry Slim w. yogurt	95
Healthy Balance	75

	C	F
Healthy Balance w. yogurt	95	
Holy-Cal	94	
Holy-Cal w. yogurt	114	
Peachy Lean	96	
Peachy Lean w. yogurt	116	
Raspberry DeLITE	59	
Raspberry DeLITE w. yogurt	85	
Raspberry Revitalizer	79	
Raspberry Revitalizer w. yogurt	84	
Tropical Replenisher	61	
Tropical Replenisher w. yogurt	87	
Workout Whey	92	
Workout Whey w. yogurt	112	

TGI Friday's ®

	C	F
Buffalo Wings, Double Glazed, 3 pieces	2	0
Bunless Burgers, 1 order (2 patties)		6
Honey BBQ Wings, 3 pieces	5	0
Key West Grouper, 1 order		12
Mozzarella Sticks, 1 piece	7	0
Mozzarella Sticks with sauce, 1 piece	10	0.3
Potato Skins, 1 full size skin (about 3 pieces)	15	4
Potato Skins snack chips, Sour Cream & Onion flavor, about 16 chips	16	1
Santa Fe Chicken Salad		
Steak Quesadilla Rolls, 2 pieces	21	<1
Tuscan Spinach Dip with vegetables, 1 appetizer	17	

Togo's Eatery®

	C	F
SANDWICHES, REGULAR 6" ROLL	69	
Albacore Tuna	79	
Avocado & Cucumber	78	
Avocado & Turkey	64	
BBQ Beef	68	
California Chicken	70	
Cheese	93	

	C	F
Hot Pastrami	72	
Hummus	104	
Meatball	80	
Philly Cheesesteak	102	
Reuben	69	
Roast Beef	68	
The Italian	68	
Turkey & Cheese	71	
Turkey, Ham & Cheese	70	
Turkey, Roast Beef & Cheese	70	
Large Size: Add 50% to Regular Size		

SALADS

	C	F
Chicken Caesar, 9 oz	13	
Farmers Market, 9 oz	18	
Oriental Salad, 21.3 oz	53	
Taco, 24.5 oz	79	

DRESSINGS

	C	F
Caesar Dressing	9	
Low Fat Balsamic Vinaigrette	9	
Oriental Sesame Salad Dressing	15	
Ranch Dressing	3	
Sesame Orange Ginger	19	

SOUPS

	C	F
Black Bean	27	
Chicken Noodle, Chili, average	20	
New England Clam Chowder	6	

Uno Chicago Grill®

ENTREES

	C	F
Tomato Basil Chicken	83	
Veggie Burger Meal	104	
Zesty Pasta Marinar	75	

THIN CRUST 9" INDIVIDUAL PIZZA

	C	F
Vegetarian: w. Cheese	127	
Vegetarian: w/o Cheese	124	

SOUP, SALAD, VEGES

	C	F
Light Lunch w. Salad	141	
Light Lunch w. Soup	150	

	C	F
Pasta Green Salad	69	
Special House	17	
Tomato Garden Vegetable	25	
Veggie Dip Platter	77	

WAWA®

BREAKFAST ITEMS

	C	F
Bagel: Plain	61	
Bagel: w. Butter	64	
Bagel: w. Cream Cheese	66	
Bagel: average, other varieties	66	
Breakfast Bowls: Creamed Chipped Beef on a Biscuit	45	
Breakfast Bowls: Sausage Gravy on a Biscuit	43	
Croissant: regular, 2 oz	35	
Hash Brown: 1, 1.7oz	10	
Muffins: Banana Walnut, 4 oz	48	
Muffins: Blueberry, 4.2 oz	55	
Muffins: Chocolate Chip, 4 oz	52	
Muffins: Corn, 4oz	55	
Sizzli Bagels: Bacon Egg Sausage & Cheese	53	
Sizzli Bagels: Sausage Egg & Cheese	54	
Sizzli Biscuits: Bacon Egg Sausage & Cheese	37	
Sizzli Biscuits: Sausage Egg & Cheese	37	
Sizzli Muffins: Bacon Egg & Cheese	31	
Sizzli Muffins: Sausage & Egg	31	

HOT SANDWICHES (NO CHEESE UNLESS INDICATED)

	C	F
Hot Sandwiches: BBQ Pork Kaiser	61	
Hot Sandwiches: Chicken Breaded Club	56	
Classics: BBQ Pork w. Cheese	112	
Classics: Chicken Grilled, no Dressing	40	
Classics: Meatball w. Cheese	49	
Classics: Roast Beef Homestyle w/ Cheese	67	
Bagel Melts: Ham & Cheese	67	
Bagel Melts: Pepperoni & Cheese	67	
Bagel Melts: Turkey Club w. Mayo	70	

COLD SANDWICHES (NO CHEESE UNLESS INDICATED)

	C	F
Italian w. Pesto & Roasted Peppers	40	
Pepper Turkey & Roasted Tomato	41	
Roast Beef & Horseradish	26	
Healthy Choice: Chicken on White	27	
Healthy Choice: Ham on White	28	
Healthy Choice: Smoked Turkey on White	31	
Healthy Choice: Roast Beef on White	31	
Turkey Carolina on White, average	30	
Turkey on White	67	
Roast Beef	37	
Seafood Salad	46	
Tuna Salad	43	
Veggie	37	
Veggie Supreme	43	

COLD SHORTIES

	C	F
American	40	
BLT, Cheese, average	37	
Chicken Salad	41	
Egg Salad w. Cheese	43	
Healthy Choice: Ham, Roast Beef	40	
Healthy Choice: Honey Smoked Turkey	42	

HOT SHORTIES

	C	F
Chicken Grilled	42	
Meatball w. Cheese	49	
Roast Beef Homestyle w. Cheese	40	

WRAPS

	C	F
Buffalo Blue Chicken	33	
Roast Beef & Pepper Jack	42	
Roasted Chicken Caesar	33	
Smoked Turkey Supreme	44	
Turkey Bacon & Colby Jack	37	

HOT DOGS

	C	F
¼ lb Beef Frank	20	

	C	F
All Beef Hot Dog	20	
Big Bacon Cheese Dog	37	
Hot Sausage	21	
Kielbasa	21	

BOWLS: PER 12 OZ BOWL

	C	F
Chicken Teriyaki	94	
Chili	86	
Steak & Vegetable	46	
Southwest Chicken	82	

SIDES: PER MEDIUM (11 OZ)

	C	F
Beef Stew	24	
Chili	31	
Homestyle Chicken & Noodles	26	
Macaroni & Cheese	45	
Mashed Potatoes	49	
Meatballs in a Cup	14	
Shepherd's Pie	37	

SOUPS: PER MEDIUM (11 OZ)

	C	F
Boston Clam Chowder	26	
Chicken Corn Chowder	29	
Potato Au Gratin	40	
Potato w. Bacon	25	

DRINKS (PER 12 OZ)

	C	F
Cappuccino	27	
French Vanilla	30	
Fat Free Cappuccino	37	
Frozen Cappuccino	47	

Wendy's®

SANDWICHES & MEALS

	C	F
Chicken Breast Fillet, No Bun, Breaded, 1 piece	13	0
Chicken Breast Fillet, No Bun, Grilled, 1 piece	1	0
Chicken Club Sandwich, 1 each	47	2
Chicken Fillet Homestyle or Spicy Sandwich, 1 each	57	2
Chicken Fillet, Spicy, No bun, 1 piece	16	0
Chicken Nuggets, 10 pieces	25	0

	C	F
Chicken Strips, Homestyle, 3 pieces	33	0
Chicken, Crispy, Sandwich, 1 each	43	1
Chicken, Grilled, Sandwich, 1 each	36	2
Classic Big Bacon Burger, 1 each	46	3
Classic Single® with Everything, 1 each	37	2
Fish Sandwich, 1 each	50	2
Frescata Sandwiches, average	51	4
Hamburger Patty, 2 oz patty	0	0
Hamburger Patty, Quarter Pound (8 oz) patty	0	0
Jr. Burgers, Any Variety, average	35	2
Kids' Meal, Any Burger, or Any Sandwich, 1 meal	33	2
Kids' Meal, Crispy Chicken Nuggets™, 4 pieces	9	0
Kids' Meal, Crispy Chicken Nuggets™, 5 pieces	11	0
Ultimate Chicken Grill Sandwich, 1 each	44	2

DRESSINGS & SAUCES

	C	F
Barbecue Sauce, 1 pkt	10	0
Blue Cheese Dressing, 1 pkt	3	0
Buffalo Sauce, 1 each	46	3
French Dressing, 1 pkt	13	0
French, Fat Free Dressing, 1 pkt	18	0
Honey Mustard Dressing, 1 pkt	11	0
Honey Mustard Dressing, low fat, 1 pkt	21	0
Honey Mustard Sauce, 1 pkt	6	0
Italian Caesar Dressing, 1 pkt	1	0
Italian Vinaigrette Dressing, 1 pkt	9	0
Italian, Reduced Fat Dressing, 1 pkt	6	0
Oriental Sesame Dressing, 1 pkt	21	0
Ranch Dressing, Hidden Valley® Reg or Reduced Fat, 1 pkt.	5	0
Ranch, Buffalo Dipping Sauce	2	0
Ranch, Heartland Dipping Sauce, 1 pkt	1	0
Spicy Southwest Chipolte Sauce, 1 pkt	5	0
Sweet & Sour Sauce, 1 pkt	12	0

	C	F
Sweet & Spicy Hawaiian Dipping Sauce, 1 pkt	17	0
Thousand Island Dressing, 1 pkt	8	0

POTATOES & FRIES

	C	F
French Fries, kids, 3.2 oz	37	3
French Fries, medium, 5.0 oz	58	5
French Fries, Biggie®, 5.6 oz	64	6
French Fries, Great Biggie®, 6.7 oz	77	7
Hot Stuffed Baked Potato™, Plain, app. 10 oz	61	7
Hot Stuffed Baked Potato™, Bacon & Cheese, 1	78	7
Hot Stuffed Baked Potato™, Broccoli & Cheese, 1	80	9
Hot Stuffed Baked Potato™, Sour Cream & Chive, 1	63	7
Potato Chips, Baked Lays, 1 bag	26	2

INDIVIDUAL ITEMS

	C	F
American Cheese, 1 slice	0	0
Bacon, 1 piece	0	0
Cheddar Cheese, Shredded, 2 tbsp	1	0
Honey Mustard, Reduced Calorie, 1 tsp	2	0
Kaiser Bun, 1 each	38	1
Ketchup, 1 tsp	2	0
Lettuce, 1 leaf	0	0
Mayonnaise, 1.5 tsp	1	0
Mustard, 0.5 tsp	0	0
Onions, 4 rings	1	0
Pickles, 4 slices	0	0
Saltine Crackers, 2 each	4	0
Sandwich Bun, 1 each	31	1
Soft Breadstick, 1 each	23	1
Taco Chips, 15 each	28	2
Tomatoes, 1 slice	1	0
Buttery Best Spread or Whipped Margarine, 1 pkt.	0	0
Croutons, Homestyle Garlic, 1 pkt	9	0
Almonds, Roasted, 1 pkt	4	2
Crispy Noodles, 1 pkt	10	0
Mandarin Orange Cup, 5 oz	19	1

	C	F
Yogurt, low fat Strawberry, 1 each	27	0
Granola Topping, 1 pkt	15	1

CHILI & SALADS

	C	F
Chili, small, 8 oz	23	5
Chili, large, 12 oz	35	8
Caesar Side Salad, 1 each	3	2
Deluxe Garden Salad, 1 each	10	4
Grilled Chicken Salad, 1 each	10	4
Side Salad, 1 each	8	2
Southwest Taco Salad, 1 each	32	9
Mandarin Chicken Salad, 1 each	18	3
Chicken Caesar Salad, 1 each	9	4
Chicken BLT Salad, 1 each	12	4

BEVERAGES

	C	F
1% low fat chocolate milk, 8 oz	28	0
2% reduced fat milk, 8 oz	13	0
Coca-Cola, kids	22	
Coca-Cola, value	30	
Coca-Cola, small	37	
Coca-Cola, medium	60	
Coca-Cola, large	78	
Coco-Cola, Diet, any size	0	0
Coffee, Decaf, any size	0	0
Coffee, regular, any size	1	0
Dr. Pepper, kids	21	
Dr. Pepper, value	27	
Dr. Pepper, small	34	
Dr. Pepper, medium	55	
Dr. Pepper, large	72	
Hot Cocoa, small	23	1
Hot Tea, small	0	0
Minute Maid® Light, any size		
Sprite, kids,	20	
Sprite, value	27	
Sprite, small	34	
Sprite, medium	54	
Sprite, large	71	
Sweetened Iced Tea, kids	14	
Sweetened Iced Tea, value	19	

	C	F
Sweetened Iced Tea, small	23	
Sweetened Iced Tea, medium	37	
Sweetened Iced Tea, large	49	

MR FROSTY™ ITEMS

	C	F
Frosty™, junior, 6 oz	26	0
Frosty™, small, 12 oz	56	0
Frosty™, medium, 16 oz	73	0
Fix 'n Mix Frosty™	29	0

Whataburger®

BURGERS & SANDWICHES

	C
Whataburger (1)	53
Whataburger No Bun (1)	4
Double Meat Whataburger (1)	53
Whata burger w/ Bacon/Cheese (1)	53
Triple Meat Whataburger (1)	53
Justaburger (1)	28
Whatacatch (1)	44
Whatachick'n (1)	63
Whataburger Jr. (1)	29
Grilled Chicken Sandwich w/ Dressing (1)	49
Grilled Chicken Sandwich w/ Dressing No Bun (1)	10
Grilled Chicken Fajita Taco (1)	35

WHATABURGER MEALS (WITH DRINK & FRIES)

Whataburger Meal	169
Whataburger w. Bacon &Cheese	170
Chicken Strips w. Toast & Gravy	127
Double Meat Whataburger	169
Grilled Chicken Sandwich Meal	165
WhataChick'N Sandwich Meal	172

SIDES

French Fries: small	33
French Fries: medium	50
French Fries: large	66
Onion Rings: medium	23
Onion Rings: large	35

CHICKEN & SALADS

	C	F
Chicken Strips (2)	22	
Chicken Strips Salad	29	
Chicken Strips Salad w/Cheddar Cheese, No Bacon	32	
Garden Salad	10	
Garden Salad w/Cheddar Cheese	10	
Grilled Chicken Salad	18	
Grilled Chicken Salad w/Cheddar Cheese	18	

DRESSINGS

Ranch, 2 oz	3
Ranch, Reduced Fat 2 oz	6
Low Fat Vinaigrette, 2 oz	6
Thousand Island, 2 oz	11

SHAKES

Chocolate, Strawberry: small, 20 floz	100
Chocolate, Strawberry: medium, 32 floz	146
Vanilla: small, 20 fl oz	81
Vanilla: medium. 32 fl oz	122

BREAKFAST

Bacon, 2 slices	0
Cinnamon Roll (1)	126
Hashbrown Sticks (4)	16
Texas Toast, 1 slice	42
Biscuit: Buttermilk (1)	34
Biscuit: Buttermilk w/Bacon (1)	34
Biscuit: Buttermilk w/Bacon, Egg, Cheese (1)	35
Biscuit: Buttermilk w/Egg & Cheese (1)	35
Biscuit: Buttermilk w/Sausage (1)	34
Biscuit: Buttermilk w/Sausage Gravy (1)	47
Biscuit: Buttermilk w/Sausage, Egg, Cheese (1)	35
Breakfast-On-A-Bun: w/Bacon (1)	28
Breakfast-On-A-Bun: w/Sausage (1)	28
Breakfast-On-A-Bun: Ranchero w/Bacon (1)	29

	C	F
Breakfast-On-A-Bun: Ranchero w/Sausage (1)	29	
Breakfast Platters (Biscuit/Eggs/ Hash Brown) w/Bacon (1)	52	
Breakfast Platters (Biscuit/Eggs/ Hash Brown) w/Sausage (1)	51	
Pancakes: Plain (3)	117	
Pancakes: w. Bacon, 2 slices	118	
Pancakes: w. Sausage, 1 patty	118	
Taquito: Bacon & Egg (1)	25	
Taquito: Potato & Egg (1)	33	
Taquito: Sausage & Egg (1)	25	

DESSERTS

	C	F
Hot Apple Pie 1 slice	31	
Chocolate Chunk Cookie, 2 oz	33	
White Choc Macadamia Cookie 2 oz	30	

White Castle®

SANDWICHES & HAMBURGERS

	C	F
Bacon Cheeseburger	13	
Cheeseburger	13	
Chicken Ring Sandwich	17	
Double Bacon Cheeseburger	20	
Double Cheeseburger	19	
Double White Castle	19	
Fish w. Cheese	18	
White Castle Burger	13	

SIDES

	C	F
Chicken Rings, 6 rings	16	
French Fries, small, 3.6 oz	37	
Mozzarella Cheese Sticks, 3 sticks	22	
Onion Rings, small, 1.9 oz	28	

DRINKS

	C	F
Coca-Cola, 1 6 fl oz	54	
Chocolate/Vanilla Shake, 16 fl oz	40	
Iced Tea, 16 fl oz	24	

Wings to Go®

WINGS

	C	F
Chicken Wings, Bone-In, 10 wings	0	0
Chicken Wings, Boneless, 10 wings	3.6	0.2

SAUCES

	C	F
BBQ Sauce, 2 tbsp	9	0
Buffalo Garlic Sauce, 2 tbsp	0.8	0
Cajun Sauce, 2 tbsp	2	0
Curry Sauce, 2 tbsp	0.5	0
Extra Hot Sauce, 2 tbsp	1.6	0
Golden Garlic Sauce, 2 tbsp	20	0
Homicide Sauce, t tbsp	2	<1
Honey Mustard Sauce, 2 tbsp	11	0
Hot Sauce, 2 tbsp	2	0
Lemon Pepper Sauce, 2 tbsp	0.5	0
Medium Sauce, 2 tbsp	2	0
Mild Sauce, 2 tbsp	1	0
Suicide Sauce, 2 tbsp	1	0
Sweet & Sour Sauce, 2 tbsp	10	0
Teriyaki Sauce, 2 tbsp	10	0

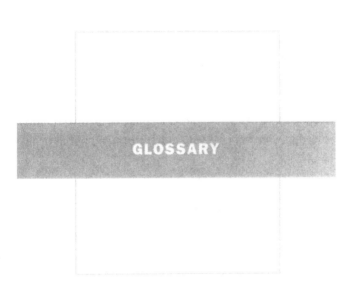

GLOSSARY

Acesulfame-K: A noncaloric artificial sweetener that is two hundred times sweeter than table sugar. It contributes no calories and does not raise blood sugar levels.

Artificial sweetener: A man-made chemical substance used to enhance the sweetness of food.

Aspartame: A low-calorie artificial sweetener commercially known as NutraSweet. It is made from two protein components (amino acids) and a trace amount of methanol, and is 180 times sweeter than table sugar. Aspartame is very low in calories and does not raise blood sugar levels.

Branched-chain starch: Complex carbohydrates composed primarily of glucose molecules loosely attached at a variety of angles and configurations. Branched-chain starches tend to digest rapidly and cause a quick rise in blood glucose levels.

Calories: Calories represent the energy content of food. Each calorie represents the heat energy required to raise 1 gram of water by 1°C.

Carb counting: The process of quantifying the amount of carbohydrate in a given food portion or complete meal or snack.

Carb factor: The percentage of a food's weight that is carbohydrate. Multiplying the food's weight (in grams) by its carb factor will yield the grams of carbohydrate.

Carbohydrate gram counting: The process of quantifying the number of grams of carbohydrate in a given food portion or complete meal or snack.

Carbohydrates: A calorie-containing organic nutrient composed of one or more sugar molecules.

Cholesterol: A steroid molecule carried in the bloodstream in the form of lipoprotein. Cholesterol is essential to the formation of bile acids, vitamin D, and a variety of hormones. When present in excessive amounts, cholesterol can contribute to blood vessel diseases.

Complex carbohydrates: Calorie-containing organic nutrients containing multiple sugar molecules. Starch, glycogen, and fiber are all forms of complex carbohydrates.

Dextrose: A simple sugar composed of two glucose molecules.

Erythritol: An artificial sweetener classified as a sugar alcohol. Erythritol has about half the calorie content and blood sugar-raising effect of ordinary sugars. Its rate of digestion is much slower than most ordinary sugars.

Exchange system: A method for organizing food according to nutritional properties. Foods within an exchange grouping have similar amounts of protein, fat, and carbohydrate.

Fiber: A form of complex carbohydrate that passes through the human digestive tract without being digested. Fiber contributes neither calories nor a rise in blood sugar levels.

Fructose: A simple 1-molecule sugar commonly found in fruit.

Galactose: A simple 1-molecule sugar that is usually combined with glucose to form lactose (milk sugar).

Glucose: A simple 1-molecule sugar absorbed rapidly into the bloodstream. Sometimes known as blood sugar or grape sugar, glucose serves as the primary energy source for most of the body's cells.

Glycemic index: A system for ranking foods according to their impact on blood sugar levels. Foods with a high glycemic index value tend to raise the blood sugar quickly; foods with a low value tend to raise the blood sugar slowly or gradually.

Glycerin: Derived from fats, glycerin is used as an additive in many diet foods. It has some of the same chemical properties as carbohydrates (including caloric content), but it does not raise blood sugar levels.

Glycerine: Another name for *Glycerin*.

Glycerol: Another name for *Glycerin*.

Glycogen: A dense storage form of complex carbohydrate found in liver and muscle cells.

Hydrogenated Starch Hydrosylates (HSH): A family of bulk artificial sweeteners that blends well with other sweeteners. Specific HSHs include glucose syrup, maltitol syrup, and sorbitol syrup. Classified as a sugar alcohol, HSH has about half the caloric content and blood sugar-raising effect of ordinary sugars. Its rate of digestion is much slower than most ordinary sugars.

Hypoglycemia: A state of low blood sugar. By definition, it is usually considered to be a blood sugar of less than 70 mg/dl.

Insoluble Fiber: A form of fiber that does not dissolve at all during digestion. Its caloric content and effect on blood sugar is negligible.

Isomalt: A bulking agent and artificial sweetener. Classified as a sugar alcohol, isomalt is 40 percent as sweet as table sugar. It has half the caloric content and blood sugar-raising effect of ordinary sugars. Its rate of digestion is much slower than most ordinary sugars.

Lactitol: A bulk artificial sweetener often blended with other low-calorie sweeteners. Classified as a sugar alcohol, lactitol is 40 percent as sweet as table sugar. It has half the caloric content and blood sugar-raising effect of ordinary sugars. Its rate of digestion is much slower than most ordinary sugars.

Lactose: A simple sugar found in milk and many other dairy products. It is composed of a glucose molecule and a galactose molecule linked together.

Maltitol: An artificial sweetener classified as a sugar alcohol. Maltitol has about half the caloric content and blood sugar-raising effect of ordinary sugars. Its rate of digestion is much slower than most ordinary sugars.

Maltose: A simple sugar composed of two glucose molecules linked together. It is sometimes known as malt sugar.

Mannitol: An artificial sweetener classified as a sugar alcohol. Mannitol has about half the caloric content and blood sugar-raising effect of ordinary sugars. Its rate of digestion is much slower than most ordinary sugars.

Portion estimation: A process by which the size of a food portion is approximated by comparing it to a standard serving size, such as one cup.

Saccharin: An artificial sweetener that passes through the body unchanged, contributing neither calories nor blood sugar.

Serving size: The amount of food typically eaten at a meal or snack. It is a standard amount determined by the government (the United States Department of Agriculture, for example) for purposes of appropriate food labeling and portion control.

Simple sugar: Calorie-containing organic nutrients containing one or two sugar molecules. Glucose, fructose, galactose, sucrose, lactose, and maltose are all types of simple sugar.

Soluble fiber: A form of fiber that dissolves partially during digestion. However, its caloric content and effect on blood sugar is negligible.

Sorbitol: A bulk artificial sweetener. Classified as a sugar alcohol, sorbitol is 60 percent as sweet as table sugar. It has about half the caloric content and blood sugar-raising effect of ordinary sugars. Its rate of digestion is much slower than most ordinary sugars.

Starch: A digestible form of complex carbohydrate composed primarily of glucose molecules.

Straight-Chain Starch: Complex carbohydrates composed of many glucose molecules attached in a linear fashion. Straight-chain starches tend to digest and raise the blood sugar more slowly than branched-chain starches.

Sucralose: Known commercially as Splenda, sucralose is a sweetening ingredient made from table sugar (sucrose). It is six hundred times sweeter than table sugar. It is very low in calories and has no effect on blood sugar.

Sucrose: A simple sugar composed of a glucose molecule and a fructose molecule linked together. It is better known as "table sugar."

Sugar: See *Simple Sugar*. For product-packaging purposes, "sugar" is often synonymous with "sucrose" or "table sugar."

Sugar alcohol: An artificial sweetener that contains approximately half the caloric content and blood sugar-raising effect of ordinary sugars. Its rate of digestion is much slower than most ordinary sugars.

Triglyerides: The form most fats take when circulating in the bloodstream. Triglycerides are composed of three fatty acid chains linked together by glycerol, a small "backbone" molecule.

Xylitol: An artificial sweetening agent that may aid in the prevention of dental cavities. Classified as a sugar alcohol, xylitol has approximately half the caloric content and blood sugar-raising effect of ordinary sugars. Its rate of digestion is much slower than most ordinary sugars.

ACKNOWLEDGMENTS

NOT BEING A dietitian myself, I have had to rely heavily on the expertise and direction of others to acquire the skills necessary to put this book together. In particular, the dietitian (and fellow Type-1 diabetic) at my practice, Judy Tripathi, has been a tremendous source of both information and confidence. If she doesn't know the answer, she always knows where to find it! My office manager, Debbie Liebman, does an incredible job of keeping twelve balls in the air at one time so that I can concentrate on one at a time. Also, thank you to Carol Tierney for her relentless diligence in helping to put the carb listings together—a task I could never have completed on my own without heavy sedation.

Outside of my practice, I wish to thank Karmeen Kulkarni and Marion Franz, two of the most talented and creative dietitians I have ever met, for always being there to answer my more challenging questions. My sincerest appreciation also goes to John Walsh (aka the Godfather of Pump

Therapy) for inspiring me (and others) to organize and educate. And thank you to Jennie Brand-Miller for her tireless work and perseverance in the study of the Glycemic Index.

Finally, my sincerest apologies to every dietitian and diabetes educator I ever met with (as a client) for fighting and questioning everything you told me to do regarding my diet. It took 20 years, but I'm finally beginning to get the point.

INDEX

The Marlowe Diabetes Library
Good control is in your hands.

MARLOWE DIABETES LIBRARY titles are available from on-line and bricks-and-mortar retailers nationally. For more information about the Marlowe Diabetes Library or any of our books or authors, visit www.marlowepub.com/diabetes library or e-mail us at goodcontrol@avalonpub.com

THE FIRST YEAR®—TYPE 2 DIABETES
An Essential Guide for the Newly Diagnosed, 2nd edition
Gretchen Becker I Foreword by Allison B. Goldfine, MD ■ $16.95

PREDIABETES
What You Need to Know to Keep Diabetes Away
Gretchen Becker I Foreword by Allison B. Goldfine, MD ■ $14.95

THE NEW GLUCOSE DIABETES REVOLUTION
The Definitive Guide to Managing Diabetes and Prediabetes Using the Glycemic Index
Dr. Jennie Brand-Miller, Kaye Foster-Powell,
Dr. Stephen Colagiuri, Alan Barclay ■ $16.95
(Coming Spring 2007)

THE NEW GLUCOSE DIABETES REVOLUTION LOW GI GUIDE TO DIABETES
The Quick Reference Guide to Managing Diabetes Using the Glycemic Index
Dr. Jennie Brand-Miller and Kaye Foster-Powell
with Johanna Burani ■ $6.95

THE 7 STEP DIABETES FITNESS PLAN
Living Well and Being Fit with Diabetes, No Matter Your Weight
Sheri R. Colberg, PhD I Foreword by Anne Peters, MD ■ $15.95

EATING FOR DIABETES
A Handbook and Cookbook—with More than 125 Delicious, Nutritious
Recipes to Keep You Feeling Great and Your Blood Glucose in Check
Jane Frank ■ $15.95

TYPE 1 DIABETES
A Guide for Children, Adolescents, Young Adults—and Their
Caregivers
Ragnar Hanas, MD, PhD | Forewords by Stuart Brink, MD,
and Jeff Hitchcock ■ $24.95

KNOW YOUR NUMBERS, OUTLIVE YOUR DIABETES
Five Essential Health Factors You Can Master to
Enjoy a Long and Healthy Life
Richard A. Jackson, MD, and Amy Tenderich ■ $14.95

INSULIN PUMP THERAPY DEMYSTIFIED
An Essential Guide for Everyone Pumping Insulin
Gabrielle Kaplan-Mayer | Foreword by
Gary Scheiner, MS, CDE ■ $15.95

1,001 TIPS FOR LIVING WELL WITH DIABETES
Firsthand Advice that Really Works
Judith H. McQuown | Foreword by Harry Gruenspan, MD, PhD $16.95

DIABETES ON YOUR OWN TERMS
Janis Roszler, RD, CDE, LD/N ■ $14.95

THINK LIKE A PANCREAS
A Practical Guide to Managing Diabetes with Insulin
Gary Scheiner, MS, CDE | Foreword by Barry Goldstein, MD ■ $15.95

THE ULTIMATE GUIDE TO ACCURATE CARB COUNTING
Gary Scheiner, MS, CDE ■ $9.95

THE MIND-BODY DIABETES REVOLUTION
A Proven New Program for Better Blood Sugar Control
Richard S. Surwit, PhD, with Alisa Bauman ■ $14.95